Bulimia / *Anorexia*

Bulimia / *Anorexia*

THE BINGE / PURGE CYCLE

AND SELF-STARVATION

Marlene Boskind-White, Ph.D.

William C. White, Jr., Ph.D.

W · W · NORTON & COMPANY *New York   London*

The text and display of this book are composed in Adobe Garamond
Composition by Allentown Digital Services Division of RR Donnelly & Sons Company
Manufacturing by Haddon Craftsmen Inc.

Library of Congress Cataloging-in-Publication Data

Boskind-White, Marlene.
  Bulimia/anorexia : the binge/purge cycle and self-starvation / Marlene Boskind-White,
  William C. White, Jr.—[3rd ed.].
      p. cm.
  Rev. ed. of: Bulimarexia. 2nd ed. 1987.
  Includes bibliographical references and index.
  ISBN 0-393-04841-1
  1. Bulimia. 2. Anorexia nervosa. 3. Women—Mental health. 4. Eating disorders.
  I. White, William C., Jr. II. Boskind-White, Marlene. Bulimarexia. III. Title.

RC552.B84 B67 2000
616.85'263—dc21
                                                                99-045784

W. W. Norton & Company, Inc., 500 Fifth Avenue, New York, N.Y. 10110
www.wwnorton.com

W. W. Norton & Company Ltd., 10 Coptic Street, London WC1A 1PU

1 2 3 4 5 6 7 8 9 0

To my beloved husband
William C. White, Jr.
1940–1998

Contents

Preface to the Third Edition

"BULIMAREXIA," the binge/purge syndrome, was introduced to the professional and popular literature in a series of articles William C. White, Jr. and I published in the 1970s. At that time during our initial research at Cornell University, the diagnostic category "bulimia" was described as a rare disorder that involved binge eating with no reference to purging and, like anorexia nervosa, was overwhelmingly interpreted and managed within the boundaries of psychoanalytic theory. Many of the young women who responded to our initial outreach efforts had been previously labeled anorexic by therapists, and most found the clinical description of the emaciated anorexic foreign and frightening. This diagnosis seemed inappropriate for women whose weights were within normal ranges and who were not starving themselves. Rather, these women were bingeing on copious quantities of food and purging themselves via forced vomiting, laxatives, diuretics, constant dieting, and/or excessive exercise.

Bulimarexia distinguished the binge/purge cycle from bulimia and anorexia nervosa. We also chose the new word to better reflect our view that binge/purge practices represented tenacious habits, not disease processes. We believed bingeing and purging were learned behaviors that could be unlearned, utilizing the principles of social learning theory. Bulimarexia was thus defined in terms of specific primary and secondary behaviors. This definition became commensurate with the revised third edition of the *American Psychiatric Association: Diagnostic and Statistical Manual of Mental*

Disorders, and the terms *bulimia nervosa* and *bulimarexia* have come to be used interchangeably. In this new edition of *Bulimarexia* I have changed the book's title to reflect the new accepted wider meaning of "bulimia" as well as the inclusion of new material on anorexia but to minimize resetting have retained the term "bulimarexia" in the original text. In the 1994 Fourth Edition of the *DSM,* the diagnostic criteria for anorexia nervosa and bulimia nervosa were revised as follows:

307.1 *Anorexia Nervosa*

A. Refusal to maintain body weight at or above a minimally normal weight for age and height (e.g., weight loss leading to maintenance of body weight less than 85 percent of that expected or failure to make expected weight gain during period of growth, leading to body weight less than 85 percent of that expected).
B. Intense fear of gaining weight or becoming fat, even though underweight.
C. Disturbance in the way in which one's body weight or shape is experienced, undue influence of body weight or shape on self-evaluation, or denial of the seriousness of the current low body weight.
D. In postmenarcheal females, amenorrhea; i.e., the absence of at least three consecutive menstrual cycles. (A woman is considered to have amenorrhea if her periods occur only following hormone, e.g., estrogen, administration.)

Specify type:
Restricting Type: during the current episode of Anorexia Nervosa, the person has not regularly engaged in binge eating or purging behavior (i.e., self-induced vomiting or the misuse of laxatives, diuretics, or enemas).
Binge-Eating/Purging Type: during the current episode of Anorexia Nervosa, the person has regularly engaged in binge eating or purging behavior (i.e., self-induced vomiting or the misuse of laxatives, diuretics, or enemas).

307.51 *Bulimia Nervosa*

A. Recurrent episodes of binge eating. An episode of binge eating is characterized by both of the following:

(1)   eating, in a discrete period of time (e.g., within any two-hour period), an amount of food that is definitely larger than most people would eat during a similar period of time and under similar circumstances

(2)   a sense of lack of control over eating during the episode (e.g., a feeling that one cannot stop eating or control what or how much one is eating)

B.   Recurrent inappropriate compensatory behavior in order to prevent weight gain, such as self-induced vomiting; misuse of laxatives, diuretics, enemas, or other medications; fasting; or excessive exercise.

C.   The binge eating and inappropriate compensatory behaviors both occur, on average, at least twice a week for three months.

D.   Self-evaluation is unduly influenced by body shape and weight.

E.   The disturbance does not occur exclusively during episodes of Anorexia Nervosa.

Specify type:

Purging Type: During the current episode of Bulimia Nervosa, the person has regularly engaged in self-induced vomiting or the misuse of laxatives, diuretics, or enemas.

Nonpurging Type: During the current episode of Bulimia Nervosa, the person has used other inappropriate compensatory behaviors, such as fasting or excessive exercise, but has not regularly engaged in self-induced vomiting or the misuse of laxatives, diuretics, or enemas.

From the outset we were dismayed and astonished at the tremendous response to our publications. Thousands of women responded to our early work, readily revealing their binge/purge behavior. Their pain and shame were overwhelming as they bemoaned their wasted talents, interrupted relationships, and significant medical problems. The first edition of our book took five years to write. Without the hundreds of bulimarexic clients who educated us during that time, it never would have happened. The book is theirs—a tribute to their trials and tribulations. From their strengths and moments of weakness, much valuable learning emerged. We are proud to have known and worked with these women and want to acknowledge their enormous talent and potential. Although the accounts they contributed are true, in every case we have changed their names and other details in order to protect their identities.

When the first edition was finally published in 1983, its reception surpassed our wildest expectations. Once again we received thousands of letters from women, thanking us and telling us that the book had given them hope. After reading it, many were able to reach out to therapy for the first time knowing that they were not alone, help was available, and success was possible. A significant number of women wrote that they had curtailed their binge/purge cycle on the basis of the book itself, without therapy. The self-help insights and strategies we outlined had helped them help themselves. Professionals wrote to us as well, and parents of bulimarexics thanked us for what they felt was the first compassionate treatment of their responsibilities and concerns.

It soon became clear to us that a second edition would be necessary. As the years passed, we began to realize that bulimarexia posed a growing health threat. We talked about these alarming medical findings in the second edition as well as including important information on nutritional counseling and strategies for learning to eat normally. The second edition also addressed our view that an overemphasis on pharmacological treatment was dangerous and demeaning to women—from a medical, psychological, and feminist point of view. We had become extremely concerned over what we felt was an attempt to medicate away a psychosocial disorder in a population that had dramatically demonstrated a vulnerability to addictive behaviors. We added a new chapter on one-to-one psychotherapy with bulimarexics, with information on group, family, and couple counseling. We discussed preventive as well as model eating-disorder programs in schools and on college campuses.

Yet after more than ten years, eating disorders had not significantly declined. On the contrary, the brightest and the best of young American women continued to overwhelm my private practice. These dutiful daughters and high achievers now included not only bulimarexics but increasing numbers of starving children, adolescents, and college-age women. Sick, pale, their skin stretched over their skulls with sunken and black-circled eyes, they were obsessed with losing weight. Anorexia had become a battle between a starving body and dying self-esteem. I realized I would need to learn more about how to treat these starving girls. Both bulimarexics and anorexics are obsessed with their weight, but bulimarexics believe they can't stop eating and anorexics won't start. Bulimarexics usually maintain a normal weight, while anorexics lose up to 25 percent of their body weight. Experts estimate that as many as one-half of all anorexics may eventually develop bulimarexia. When they no longer can maintain starving they employ purging practices.

I approached the writing of this new edition with deep sorrow because of the devastating tragic loss of my best friend, coauthor, partner, and soul mate, Bill, who was killed in an automobile accident on April 6, 1998. Norton's interest in a new third edition began to help me recover enthusiasm for my life and its direction. I became excited about writing once again because I have learned and experienced a great deal that I hope will be a valuable adjunct to what we have already written. The entire book has been enhanced and updated. For this new edition I have added chapters on the outpatient treatment of anorexia and another on managed care. The chapters on anorexia nervosa focus on the neglected sociocultural roots of this disorder, discuss outpatient treatment strategies from the first session through termination, and underline why feminist consciousness-raising needs to be legitimized, resurrected, and implemented in therapy as a powerful tool to help girls find out exactly what it means to grow up female in America.

The chapter on managed care is written for therapists treating eating disorders and offers strategies for both working with and working without managed care. It discusses practice building and niche marketing to attract self-pay clients. For those who have to work with managed care, I outline coping strategies, writing managed-care-friendly eating-disorder treatment plans, and ways to implement appeals and fight back when treatment plans are rejected.

In the final chapter, "Our Daughters, Ourselves," I offer suggestions for embarking on a new activist journey to combat cultural values that promote eating disorders. I continue to believe the girls and women I work with are not sick but are instead embryonic, lacking important tools available to males from infancy. I also have not met those terrible people called "parents"—especially mothers. Blaming mothers detracts from more important themes and perpetuates mother-daughter conflict. To the contrary, we need to break down the barriers of suspicion and distrust keeping them apart. Girls need to see that society has also oppressed their mothers and that they share commonalities of experience. They need their mothers more than ever.

Throughout this book we will be speaking of women and girls. In the past we have been criticized for neglecting the 5 percent or so of males who also grievously suffer from eating disorders. We have never written about males because we know very little about them. Over a span of twenty-five years we have treated only a handful of men. For a discussion of males with eating disorders, we refer the reader to Arnold E. Anderson, M.D., the author of *Practical Comprehensive Treatment of Anorexia Nervosa and Bulimia* (1985). He has written extensively about this subgroup of sufferers.

There are many friends and colleagues I must thank for their contributions to this new edition. All have made suggestions that have strengthened the manuscript. Dr. William Ball and Dr. Bruce Fariss have been invaluable in revising the section on medical implications. Alison Manetta, Christine Moberg, and Lorelea Buffington functioned as research assistants and provided me with many insights. Pat Young, my nutritional consultant, has been a critical part of my treatment team for over ten years, and she offered expert help in revising the sections on nutrition. Dedee Millican provided superb secretarial assistance for this new edition. Candace Watt, my editor, has been extremely supportive. Her help is greatly appreciated.

It is my husband, Bill, though, to whom I owe the most gratitude. Without him my work with eating disorders would have never began. I met him during my two-year internship in Psychological Services at Cornell University in 1974. He was a staff psychologist, and our clinic at the time was very traditional and therefore very underutilized by students. He then became director of Psychological Services. Bright, innovative, and proactive, a behaviorist by training, he was interested in offering relevant outreach programs to address the real-life problems students were struggling with. For example, he began a suicide prevention plan that became a model for many colleges and universities. I approached him with my ideas about a program for eating disorders—and the sky was the limit! He gave me complete support and autonomy. He and I remained the best of friends for three years, and then one night we fell in love and were inseparable for over two decades.

Bill loved the simple things in life, like walking his hunting dogs and seeing them point a grouse or catching a glimpse of a red fox traversing our farm or a hawk circling overhead. Every day with Bill was a first-time experience. His unbelievable enthusiasm, talent, and energy made him totally irresistible and gave me twenty-three intense, intimate, and deeply satisfying years. I am blessed to have known and loved him. He was and always will be my hero.

Special words of love and gratitude are in order for my dearest friends, Neil and Jule Dubner, Robert and Jackie Wood, and Charlie and Laraine Simpson, for supporting me, believing in me, and helping me through the process of bereavement.

We are indebted to a number of prominent social scientists and psychotherapists whose work helped immeasurably in the formulation of our research and treatment. Although our treatment does not expouse any one school, our thinking with regard to dynamic concepts and therapeutic style has been strongly influenced by the work of Alfred Adler, Albert Bandura, Eric Berne, Albert Ellis, David Burns, Aaron Beck, William Glasser, and Fritz Perls. Feminist consciousness-raising is the foundation of our work. It asserts a positive image of female energy and teaches women how to place their feelings and experiences in a political context. Betty

Friedan, Phyllis Chesler, and Stella Resnik significantly shaped the way we incorporate feminism into our therapy.

I hope the reader will forgive the inconsistent use of "I" and "we" throughout the book. It is necessary because this third edition is a sole effort while the first two editions were written by the two of us.

M.B.W.

Bulimia / *Anorexia*

1 .

The Evolution of This Book

ON an early autumn evening in 1975, we attended a reception honoring a woman faculty member we had long admired for her scholarly, inquisitive mind and feminist philosophy. As we joined the reception line, we overheard several well-wishers applauding her latest work. We noticed that she turned aside these compliments with breezy disdain. Then a man ahead of us in line commented that she looked ravishing and seemed much slimmer than when he had last seen her. The woman beamed and replied, "That's the nicest compliment I have received all night."

As we drove home that evening, we were somewhat disillusioned and clearly sensitized by what we had observed. We were not yet aware of the complicated relationship between women and food or of the obsessional "fear of fatness" that underlies it. Soon, however, we began to see women who reminded us of this esteemed faculty friend—young, slim women who were obsessed with weight and who believed they were powerless in the face of food and that there just was too much of them. A patient named Suzanne provided our first personal insight into the problem. Marlene was beginning a two-year internship at Cornell University Psychological Services and was in a doctoral program in counseling. Suzanne had been randomly assigned to Marlene. During their second session, after an extended period of silence punctuated by tears, Suzanne blurted out: "I have a problem with food. I eat. I mean, I eat disgusting amounts of food. You can't imagine how much I eat. I go on these binges. Then I start thinking about all those calories, and . . . and I make myself throw up. I can't stop myself. I hate myself, and I don't believe I'm telling you this."

Over the next sessions a pattern began to emerge. Suzanne had been voted "most likely to succeed" in her small-town high school. Now at Cornell, a thousand miles from home, her high school A's had dwindled to C's, and she felt deeply guilty and ashamed that she was not living up to her parents' expectations, which were also her own: "They're spending so much money to send me here and I can't concentrate. Then I go out and spend their money on food and feel more guilt . . . and it goes on and on." In addition, though fashionably thin, Suzanne had had few dates; in fact, her social life lacked both male and female companionship.

Suzanne had spoken about her eating problems only once before—to a therapist she had seen while in high school. She had not, however, informed her therapist of the intensity, frequency, or duration of the binge/purge cycle that had been consuming so much of her energy. He had, therefore, reassured her by telling her that she was so thin, she need not worry about overeating. Suzanne and her therapist spent the next six months working almost exclusively on the past, exploring the issues underlying her obsession with food. Since that time she had kept her bingeing and purging a secret; she made sure that she was never caught in the act, so family and friends were not aware of her behavior. By the time she was nineteen, when she came to the clinic complaining of loneliness and depression, Suzanne had been bingeing and purging three to four times a day for six years. She had read extensively about every kind of eating disorder but had been unable to eat normally for more than a few days at a time.

Three weeks after Marlene's encounter with Suzanne, Heather, a petite, 90-pound sophomore, sought help for "heterosexual problems." She too was randomly assigned to Marlene, and she too had Suzanne's problem. "I'd rather die than be fat," she said matter-of-factly, eventually revealing that she was consuming over sixty laxatives a day after grotesque food orgies.

Within a week, Janet, a campus beauty, revealed her binge/fast cycle to Marlene, angrily blaming it on the man she loved, who had rejected her. After all-day binges, Janet starved herself for days, barely subsisting on diet pills and coffee.

After hearing these women describe such similarities in eating behavior and lifestyle, we began to question other therapists at the clinic. We learned that within the same year, each therapist had seen several patients who complained of bingeing and purging. As a rule, these patients did not initially reveal their obsession with food. Rather, they complained of depression, unsatisfying relationships, loneliness, and anxieties of one sort or another. Clearly, as a group, they were hesitant to reveal their behavior honestly, despite the emphasis within our clinic on short-term therapy, targeting specific behaviors upon which clients wished to work, and goal contracting.

We then assigned all young women who had admitted to a binge/purge problem to Marlene. Each woman had her own tale to tell, but the stories that emerged had a common theme: all involved inordinate dependency, the need for constant approval, shame and self-loathing, feelings of inadequacy and helplessness, and a terror of being "found out." In the early months of treatment, the women were unaware that Marlene was seeing others with the same complaint. In fact, they did not believe that other women were engaged in this behavior. Each felt that she had invented this bizarre habit, one so unspeakable that no one else would dream of doing it. Each lived in dread that her habit would be discovered and that she would be rejected because of it. One woman had begun to keep a diary in adolescence, around the time she began to binge and purge. Cryptic notes about her behavior appeared daily. "It's pretty bad today," she would write. "It" was never named or "owned" as something she chose to do.

Because we felt that isolation was at the center of the problem, we wanted to bring the women together for group therapy. At the same time, we suspected that there were probably other women at Cornell struggling with the same behavior who would benefit from a group experience. The rationale for initiating our pilot group therapy program gained further impetus when we discovered that twenty-six women had spontaneously revealed their binge/purge behavior to therapists at the clinic during the 1974 academic year. Without exception, they felt more desperate about and dominated by their binge/purge syndrome than by any other aspect of their lives. Nevertheless, they too had rarely discussed their obsession with food. Their sense of isolation, shame, and guilt apparently inhibited them in doing so. A follow-up questionnaire revealed that 96 percent had reverted to their former eating patterns within two months after treatment. Thus, although some had done well initially, they were consistently unable to sustain that progress, primarily because, as one woman put it, "I'm not strong enough when I need to be." It soon became clear that these women had lacked critical sources of support upon leaving therapy.

On January 15, 1975, we placed the following ad in our university newspaper:

Attention Food Bingers: For some time now you have been locked into a cycle of gorging on food and then purging either by forced vomiting, laxatives, diuretics, or continual dieting and fasting. You often feel unable to break this cycle. A group is now being started for persons struggling with this behavior pattern. If you are interested in joining us, please call this number.

We anticipated a few inquiries, but immediately received sixty-two! All but two of the respondents were women. Over the phone they sounded frightened and desperate. The respondents selected for group therapy were screened on the basis of the following operational definition of the problem:

1. The woman is locked into cyclical eating behavior. She first experiences an inordinate desire for food and then consumes vast quantities. Subsequently, she purges to get rid of the food via forced vomiting (often several times a day), fasting, constant dieting, laxative or diuretic abuse.

2. The woman exhibits a distorted body image. She complains of being too fat even though this perception is not shared by her therapist and significant others.

3. The woman complains of low self-esteem and of feelings of

inadequacy, helplessness, and despair. Often isolated, she fears rejection by men, distrusts women, and expresses great shame regarding her behavior.

OF the sixty-two subjects who responded to our advertisement, thirty-five women, nineteen to twenty-six years of age, met the above criteria. All of the women, by their own admission, had been struggling with these behaviors for several years. The mean age of onset was fifteen.

In retrospect, we realized that this first advertisement drew a response from a group of women that was more severely affected than subsequent groups we have treated. Initially the clinic was unprepared for this overwhelming response. After limiting the first group to fifteen women, we referred many women to other resources, including therapy groups at the clinic, individual therapists, and organizations such as Overeaters Anonymous. We felt compelled to treat all who wished to work with us, and, at the same time we initiated an empirical study of three different therapy groups. These studies, which were to form the basis of Marlene's dissertation, had two major purposes: (1) to obtain a more objective description of the ways in which these women differed from a comparable group of women who did not binge and purge, and (2) to evaluate the effectiveness of group treatment.

Thus we randomly assigned women to one-to-one therapy, group therapy, or a control group. Control group members were told that although the treatment group was filled, they could obtain one-to-one therapy, which we would provide immediately, or wait approximately three months to become part of the pilot therapy group. Most women who were randomly chosen for the control group decided to remain on the waiting list.

Treatment groups were led by Marlene and a female cotherapist. The group met weekly for eleven sessions. The present-centered, action-oriented thrust of contemporary psychology and behaviorism was emphasized in these groups because we believed that heightened awareness, assertiveness training, and contracting to work toward specific goals might help women overcome their persistent sense of isolation, shame, and helplessness. In addition, the therapists embraced a feminist treatment orientation in the belief that cultural factors facilitated the obsessional pursuit of slimness by socializing women to become passive, dependent, and accommodating and to value their bodies principally for physical attractiveness.

At the time of our initial research in 1975, the diagnostic category *bulimia* (from the Greek meaning "great hunger") was devoid of any reference to purging. More important, bulimia was described as a rare disorder that like anorexia (meaning to turn away from appetite), was overwhelmingly interpreted and managed within the boundaries of psychoanalytic theory. In 1955 the "Case of Laura," a slim woman who binged, was dramatized by the psychotherapist Robert Lindner in his classic book *The 50-Minute Hour*. Lindner connected Laura's oral greed with a desire to be impregnated by her father. Her "cure" necessitated an acceptance of the traditional feminine role, and Lindner's account focused on her grotesque food binges, ignoring the purging and/or starving that Laura must have engaged in in order to maintain her slim and fashionable body.

The women we were beginning to treat at Cornell found these clinical descriptions of the emaciated anorexic and the mysterious bulimic foreign and frightening and emphatically rejected psychosexual interpretations of their disorder. We decided to adopt a theroretical model that would more accurately describe this behavior and distinguish it from anorexia and bulimia. Thus, we coined the term *bulimarexia* and operationally defined this habitual behavior in terms of gorging, purging, and those salient dynamics that include perfectionism, obsessive concern with food and body proportions, isolationism, low self-esteem, and a strong commitment to please others, often at the individual's expense. Four years later, in 1979, independent researchers in England began to encounter a similar population of women who binged and purged. One clinician proposed the term "bulimia nervosa," while another chose "dietary chaos syndrome" as a means of classifying the disorder.

We did not label this disorder "bulimarexia" without considering the pitfalls in doing so. The dangers of labeling a behavioral syndrome are well known. Such labeling may legitimize a behavior as a disease process so that the "victim" need assume little or no responsibility for personal actions. Being labeled mentally ill often serves to reinforce the role of the victim and the concomitant surrender of power to a healer. We were convinced that bulimarexia was a *learned behavior,* subject to the principles of learning. Since it was learned it could be unlearned. We emphasized that the lifestyle and values adhered to by the bulimarexic were maladaptive response patterns that stemmed from the process of female socialization. It was, in our view, a process consistently reinforced by the media's "ideal female."

Over a two-year period, after carefully listening and working with over one hundred bulimarexic women, we began to develop a treatment program based upon the realities these women consistently described. Rather than a desire for oral impregnation and a rejection of femininity, the belief system and lifestyle of bulimarexics overwhelmingly suggested a deeply rooted commitment to traditional feminine values. However, it was also a commitment characterized by severe conflict. The societal pressures that contributed to bulimarexia in the women we treated were identified as the very ones that cause most women in our culture to agonize over their weight.

Marlene first presented this feminist analysis of the syndrome in an essay entitled "Cinderella's Stepsisters: A Feminist Perspective on Anorexia Nervosa and Bulimia," in the spring 1977 volume of *Signs: Journal of Women in Culture and Society.* Another article, "The Gorging-Purging Syndrome," was published in the March 1977 issue of *Psychology Today.* This article described what we had learned from our two-year intensive study of Cornell women as well as of older women from the Ithaca community and central New York.

Despite mounting interest and inquiries from women through-out the country, we still viewed the problem as a limited phe-nomenon and were unprepared for the deluge of responses this article elicited. Dozens of desperate letters began arriving daily, some ten to fifteen typewritten pages long. The women poured out the pain associated with wasted years and unfulfilled dreams. They were disillusioned, frightened, and despairing that they would ever be able to control their behavior. Many who wrote were in their late twenties and thirties. Some had been bingeing and purging for fifteen years. Others were barely in their teens: "Dr's," one began, "I am desperate and contemplating suicide because of this." One seventeen-year-old scrawled huge desperate words: "Please help me. I feel like I'm throwing up my life." All were amazed that oth-ers "did it" and were eager to know more about the problem. Most spontaneously offered to participate in our research and were eager to complete detailed questionnaires addressing a variety of famil-ial and dynamic issues.

The *Psychology Today* article eventually drew responses from over eight hundred women ranging in age from twelve to fifty-five. Equally astonishing were letters of inquiry from over one hundred professionals, many of whom were employed in college settings. They wrote that they were seeing more and more women com-plaining of this problem and requested further direction regarding treatment. Bulimarexia appeared rampant not only in colleges but also in metropolitan areas and isolated rural communities. House-wives, teenagers, and professional women were thereby added to our original population.

Early group work at Cornell proved much more productive than previous one-to-one psychotherapy in that approximately half of the group members had eliminated or significantly reduced their bingeing behavior upon six month follow up. Furthermore, the group experience was cited as critical in helping them to rec-ognize their problem and in leading them to deal with it more ac-tively. Nevertheless, these pilot treatment programs were not sufficient to alter critical aspects of the syndrome. In most cases, bingeing had reinforced abnormally low self-esteem by providing an excuse for remaining isolated and not assuming day-to-day responsibilities. The increased risk taking and the changes that occurred as a result of these groups fostered new experiences, relationships, and, therefore, new problems. Follow-up studies of these women revealed one significant feature: None of the women experienced genuine intimacy in their relationships, particularly with men. Although therapy had helped to focus on developing a sense of identity independent of men, we had apparently overlooked a major goal that was spontaneously stated by most of these women—they were eager to develop or redevelop relationships with men. The all-women groups had provided few didactic or experiential opportunities for facilitating growth in this critical area; once back in the "real world," the women, soon found an opportunity to revert to bingeing.

In the summer of 1977, after reassessing our outcome data once again, we redesigned our survey inventories and embarked upon a group therapy program that included a male therapist. Bill, in his role as director of Cornell Psychological Services, had been actively involved with the formation of the program, but so far had remained peripheral to the direct treatment of these women. In our revised therapy program, we streamlined the eleven to twelve hours of therapy provided during a college semester into a fifteen hour weekend-marathon format. The women lived and interacted with each other for the entire weekend. One half of our group time was devoted to individualized work with each woman within the context of the group. Three of the fifteen hours of treatment were conducted without Bill in order to maintain our emphasis on a feminist philosophy designed to facilitate the enhancement of a more androgynous identity. Bill's absence during these crucial hours also served to heighten a sense of honesty, risk taking, and camaraderie because it was much easier to talk about issues related to sexuality within an all-women group. Bill was, however, actively involved in the treatment process throughout the remaining twelve hours of therapy. In addition to providing many opportunities to observe important male-female transactions, group members were also able to interact directly with Bill, who served as surrogate father, boyfriend, and boss in role-plays with women who had unfinished business. Role-playing and comparable interactions provided the opportunity for women to clarify their problems with men in concrete ways, thereby helping them to acknowledge their part in relinquishing their power and perpetuating unsatisfying relationships with men. Thus, our original feminist perspective was now enhanced both by the presence of a male therapist and by the relationship training inherent in our male-female therapy team. Furthermore, the presence of a male therapist served to stimulate inquiries from fathers, husbands, brothers, and other male figures close to the lives of women in treatment. Many men were confused and angered by behavior that they were unwittingly reinforcing and consistently reached out to discuss their coping strategies with Bill. Most of them also indicated that it would have made them uncomfortable or that they would have been unwilling to express themselves in such a way to a woman therapist. From these men we received valuable insight, albeit from a different perspective, into the lives of women suffering from this secret disorder.

In August 1977 we initiated this male-female group treatment program with fourteen women who had responded to the *Psychology Today* article. Ranging in age from eighteen to forty-five, all of these women had been binge eating and purging for at least four years. Most binged daily, at least twice, and were purging one or more times during an eight-hour interval. In every case, bulimarexia was the primary maladaptive behavioral pattern. None of the women were clinically underweight or in need of medical management at the time of treatment. A letter from a physician attesting to their height, weight, and general medical condition was an admission requirement. Since this was a pilot study, we administered the California Psychological Inventory (CPI), a body cathexis test, which rates a person's feelings about different parts of their body to tap potential changes in body image and our survey inventory prior to the initiation of therapy, immediately after the group finished, and one year later. This time our results were more favorable, particularly with regard to eliminating or attenuating the bingeing behavior. Furthermore, attitude changes were noted and were accompanied by a more active, ambitious, and versatile role orientation. The one-year follow-up revealed that group participants had broadened their outlook and interests, as measured by the CPI, and no longer loathed their bodies as indicated by a significant increase in their body cathexis scores.

Feedback from questionnaires was especially valuable. For example, the women reported that they felt the group size was too large. We agreed and gradually limited it in subsequent workshops, finally realizing that eight to ten women was an appropriate number. Because of other suggestions, we discarded certain techniques that the women believed were ineffectual or detrimental. One of these involved keeping a diary of daily food intake. The women felt this merely gave them permission to obsess about food during valuable group time. They believed the group was most productive when it focused on other aspects of their lives. They were tired of talking about food!

The apparent success of this first group program encouraged us to offer others. We also began to open our workshops to professionals as a teaching forum for sharing our insights and techniques. In this way, we have been able to extend our treatment to more and more women in need of help.

In September 1979 *Glamour* magazine published an article based upon interviews with us and with former clients who had agreed to share their experiences. The response to this article was so overwhelming that *Glamour* devoted its December 1979 editorial to a discussion of the enormous response that it had received. The editorial staff was staggered by the number of women who wrote, but, more importantly, it was shocked by the desperate, often hopeless message so consistently expressed:

In September of this year, we published the article, *"Full Stomachs and Empty Lives,"* about bulimarexia, a little publicized destructive behavior pattern. . . . The reaction to this article has been startling and thought provoking—unlike any in our publishing experience—not only in the volume of mail but also in the desperate tone of many of the letters. One women described bulimarexia as "the helpless anguish, the sheer hell, in which I am drowning." "I'm not quite sure how much longer I can go on like this," wrote another, and a third woman said fatalistically, "Although suicide seemed far away, nonetheless it was ultimately the only viable solution. . . ."

The *Glamour* editorial board was especially disturbed by the secrecy and shame that intensified feelings of aloneness and despair:

Bulimarexia had been a problem for a long time, but readers who wrote us had shared it with no one. They paid the emotional toll, sometimes for years, thinking somehow that this life was all they deserved. . . . Women still hide their private terrors from the world and even from those closest to them. Over and over again the letters said, "You mean I am not alone?" "It hit me so hard I'm sitting here shaking my head. I really thought I was the only one in the world with that problem." "It is my big dark secret of which I am terribly ashamed. . . ."

In May 1980 an article on bulimarexia by Marie Brenner appeared in *Savvy: The Magazine for Executive Women.* Professional women from all walks of life—lawyers, physicians, dancers, athletes, psychologists, and business women—wrote to us and revealed that they were consumed by the same shame, isolation, and despair. They too were bulimarexics! Other articles about our work with bulimarexic women soon followed. Feature articles in *Ladies' Home Journal* and *Seventeen* brought forth another flood of responses. Alarmed and disheartened by the hundreds of letters from preteens, we began to concentrate on the preventive aspects of this disorder, with particular regard to students in high schools and universities. These outreach activities have been encouraging in that a significant number of men are attending our lectures and asking for advice about how best to deal with girlfriends and other loved ones struggling with the syndrome. Equally rewarding has been our consulting work with mental health practitioners within these institutions who are eager to learn more effective treatment and preventive techniques.

We also act as consultants to private and public high schools and have enjoyed regular speaking engagements on "Health Awareness Day" and other such occasions. Such opportunities help to fortify young women with the skills they need to deal with the precursors of bulimarexia. We expect to continue this kind of outreach activity in the future as an adjunct to our applied research and workshops, now being offered on a monthly basis at a variety of settings throughout the country.

This book was written for bulimarexic women, all of whom long to live fully but are paralyzed by shame, insecurity, and fear of rejection. Their escape from their self-imposed pain involves relinquishing control; eventually, perhaps the damage can be averted before it manifests itself. This book is also written for the myriad young women who are not yet bulimarexic but who have the foresight to recognize their vulnerability to problems with food.

We have attempted to address the concerns of families and friends directly involved with bulimarexic and prebulimarexic women, for their support—appropriately rendered—is necessary.

Finally, it is our hope that professional therapists will profit from our errors and insights and will find within these pages suggestions that will enhance their clinical skills so that they can aid those in need of intervention.

We have researched and treated over two thousand women since Suzanne first struggled with her confession, and although we have no idea how many more women are secretly engaged in this pernicious behavior, we are convinced the number is staggering. Although treatment has been arduous, the rewards have been significant. Bulimarexic women are, in general, bright, talented, and capable. Their prognosis, in our experience, is good primarily because of their strengths and because of the fact that bulimarexia is now receiving serious attention from the professional community. It is our hope that this book will further heighten awareness and will help illuminate the way to more concrete means of curtailing and eliminating this destructive habit.

2.

The Binge/Purge Cycle:
Thin Is Never Thin Enough

NICOLE awakes in her cold, dark room and already wishes it was time to go back to bed. She dreads the thought of going through this day, which will be like so many others in her recent past. She asks herself the same question every morning: "Will I be able to make it through the day without being totally obsessed by thoughts of food, or will I blow it again and spend the day bingeing?" She tells herself that today she will begin a new life, today she will start to live like a normal human being. However, she is not at all convinced that the choice is hers.

She feels fat and wants to lose weight, so she decides to start a new diet: "This time it'll be for real! I know I'll feel good about myself if I'm thinner. I want to start my exercises again because I want to make my body more attractive."

Nicole plans her breakfast but decides not to eat until she has worked out for a half hour or so. She tries not to think about food since she is not really hungry. She feels anxiety about the day ahead of her. "It's this tension," she rationalizes. That is what is making her want to eat.

Nicole showers and dresses and plans her schedule for the day—classes, studying, and meals. She plans this schedule in great detail, listing where she will be at every minute and what she will eat at every meal. She does not want to leave blocks of time when she might feel tempted to binge.

"It's time to exercise, but I don't really want to; I feel lazy. Why do I always feel so lazy? What happened to the willpower I used to have?"

Gradually, Nicole feels the bingeing signal coming on. Half-heartedly she tries to fight it, remembering the promises she made to herself about changing. She also knows how she is going to feel at the end of the day if she spends it bingeing. Ultimately, Nicole decides to give in to her urges because, for the moment, she would rather eat.

Since Nicole is not going to exercise, because she wants to eat, she decides that she might as well eat some "good" food. She makes a poached egg and toast and brews a cup of coffee, all of which goes down in about thirty seconds. She knows this is the beginning of several hours of craziness!

After rummaging through the cupboards, Nicole realizes that she does not have any binge food. It is cold and snowy outside, and she has to be at school fairly soon, but she bundles up and runs down the street. First she stops at the bakery for a bagful of sweets—cookies and doughnuts. While munching on these, she stops and buys a few bagels. Then comes a quick run to the grocery store for granola and milk. At the last minute Nicole adds several candy bars. By the time she is finished, she has spent over fifteen dollars.

Nicole can hardly believe that she is going to put all of this food, this junk, into her body; even so, her adrenaline is flowing, and all she wants to do is eat, think about eating, and anticipate getting it over with. She winces at the thought of how many pounds all of this food represents but knows she will throw it up afterward. There is no need to worry.

At home Nicole makes herself a few bowls of cereal and milk, which she gobbles down with some of the bagels smothered with butter, cream cheese, and jelly (not to mention the goodies from the bakery and the candy bars that she is still working on). She drowns all of this with huge cups of hot coffee and milk, which help speed up the process even more. All this has taken no longer than forty-five minutes, and Nicole feels as though she has been moving at ninety miles an hour.

Nicole dreads reaching this stage, where she is so full that she absolutely has to stop eating. She will throw up, which she feels she has to do but which repels her. At this point, she has to acknowledge that she's been bingeing. She wishes she were dreaming but knows all too well that this is real. The thought of actually digesting all of those calories, all of that junk, terrifies her.

In her bathroom, Nicole ties her hair back, turns on the shower (so none of the neighbors can hear her), drinks a big glass of water, and proceeds to force herself to vomit. She feels sick, ashamed, and incredulous that she is really doing this. Yet she feels trapped—she does not know how to break out of this pattern. As her stomach empties, she steps on and off the scale to make sure she has not gained any weight.

Nicole knows she needs help, but she wants someone else to make it all go away. As she crashes on her bed to recuperate, her head is spinning. "I'll never do this again," she vows. "Starting tomorrow, I'm going to change. I'll go on a fast for a week, and then I'll feel better."

Unfortunately, deep inside, Nicole does not believe any of this. She knows this will not be the last time. Reluctantly, she leaves for school, late and unwilling to face the work and responsibilities that lie ahead. She almost feels as though she could eat again to avoid going to school. She wonders how many hours it will be until she starts her next binge, and she wishes she had never gotten out of bed this morning.

Nicole has been a binger for five years. She started bingeing once a week and moved to several times a day after the first year. There were very few days when she did not binge. If she refrained, it was only because of "white knuckling it" (as she put it), which she could hardly maintain for more than a day.

The bingeing started when Nicole arrived on campus as a freshman. She gained fifteen pounds and felt alone and unable to maintain a diet. Nicole added to her isolation by choosing to live in a single dorm room. Her binges increased in frequency and duration in her junior year, when she became engaged to a medical student and moved in with him. It was Allen who jokingly suggested one night that she force herself to vomit after one of her typical "poor me" dialogues about how much she had eaten and how awful she looked. Nicole's misery and shame increased as she grew thinner and more dependent on purging to offset her binges. Allen and Nicole lived together for one year before Nicole fled the relationship for the "safety" of her family. However, since she had traded one form of dependency for another and was doing little more than hanging out at her family's home, she continued to binge and vomit. At the urging of her family, she began intensive psychotherapy, but after six months of dealing exclusively with the past, Nicole felt more hopeless and locked into the behavior than ever.

Nicole suffers from bulimarexia, a cyclical eating disorder that has reached epidemic proportions in our culture. The details of a typical day in Nicole's life are not pleasant to read about—and certainly are not pleasant to live through. Her day may differ in certain aspects from that of other bulimarexic women, but her behavior and her ways of coping with stress will be all too familiar to the thousands of women who alternately binge and then purge by self-induced vomiting, the abuse of laxatives and diuretics, or severe fasting.

Bulimarexia can affect women at any age, from the teens well into middle age. However, white middle-class adolescents and women in their twenties with a strong orientation toward academic achievement and a traditional lifestyle, including marriage, are most vulnerable. Many are highly intelligent, attractive in appearance, and capable of handling successful careers. Yet traditionally they have abnormally low self-esteem, a desire for perfection, a sense of loneliness and isolation, and an obsession with food as it relates to body weight. Some of these women feel as though they have split into two people. One is the competent woman the outside world sees; the other is the driven, out-of-control woman who will cheat, steal, or lie to satisfy her urge to binge.

In time, as the behavior increases in intensity, these women arrive at the irrational conclusion that the bulimarexic part of their personality is the "real" woman, thereby negating and undermining any successes they may experience in other aspects of their lives.

In some ways, there are similarities with anorexia nervosa, the self-starvation syndrome: the lack of self-esteem, the paralyzing sense of ineffectiveness, the distorted body image, the obsessive concern with food. Both anorexics and bulimarexics are likely to have been brought up in middle-class, upwardly mobile families, where mothers are characterized as overinvolved in their daughters' lives and fathers are preoccupied with work outside the home. For the most part, both anorexics and bulimarexics were "good children," eager to comply and achieve in order to elicit the love and approval of others.

We have, however, noted significant differences between these two groups of women. Biochemical changes that result from sustained self-starvation typically bond physiological abnormalities with psychological deficits in the anorexic. The apathy and irritability that contribute to the anorexic's unyielding stance in therapy are not as prominent among bulimarexics. Anorexics are generally younger, far less socially competent, and much more isolated from and dependent upon the family than bulimarexics. While both are obsessed with food, for anorexics eating rampages are likely to be infrequent occurrences. In sudden fits of hunger, anorexic women may binge and purge in solitude, but this is the exception rather than the rule. In fact, the anorexic is near starvation much of the time.

In contrast, the binge and purge becomes a ritual in the lives of bulimarexic women. In moments of stress, they turn *toward* food, not *away* from it. When they are able to control their behavior, they often eat highly nutritious meals in an effort to repair the harm they have done to their bodies. And for the most part they are able to function in social and work contexts, though not without difficulty. Their health may certainly be affected, but their very lives are not necessarily in danger, as is often the case with anorexics. Ultimately, we have come to view this syndrome as related to anorexia yet distinct from it.

Many women teeter on the brink of anorexia or bulimarexia during adolescence. This is the time when girls become acutely aware of other girls who seem more successful and attractive than themselves. As a result, they feel inadequate or self-conscious by comparison. In searching for "magical cures" for their existential crises, both groups—preanorexics and prebulimarexics—focus on *The Diet* as their ticket to success and happiness. What happens after this first diet is crucial and critical. Their ability to resolve the frequently unfulfilled expectations about weight loss is often dependent on support from family as well as on the life experience the young women already possess. The more isolated and locked into family they are, the greater the chance they will "choose" anorexia. Women who veer toward bulimarexia are more tenacious. They do not have to "show" their pain to the extreme evidenced in anorexia. However, their passivity and desperation and their attempts to maintain control are a matter of degree; they are, in effect, stronger carbon copies of their younger anorexic sisters.

The widespread incidence of bulimarexia has gone unrecognized until fairly recently because bingeing and purging is in essence secret behavior. These women dread the possibility that their "disgusting" habit will be revealed, and few will tell the whole story to their doctors, therapists, or families. Even when they do, professionals and well-intentioned loved ones are often unable to provide the necessary help. Many more women, unable to confess the full truth, fall back on vague hints that are typically misread. "I told my sister and mother a partial truth about throwing up sometimes after I ate, which they interpreted as nervousness," one woman said. "I was too ashamed to tell the whole truth." When they seek out professionals, too little information is forthcoming to elicit further examination or questioning. Then, too, in our society it is assumed that women are concerned about weight and vigilant about weight control. Thus, whatever halting statements bulimarexics may make are likely to be interpreted as bids for attention or attempts to elicit flattery, rather than as cries for help. The following statement is significant:

"I never mentioned this well-kept secret to my psychiatrist, except to state that I might have a problem with compulsive eating. As I was sitting in his office in my size-five dress, I'm sure he thought I was confusing an extra cookie with compulsive eating. Little did he know how adept I am at consuming a couple of family-sized packages of cookies, followed by a box of crackers, followed by three breakfast bars, followed by fifteen Ex-Lax! This is just one of many eating incidents in a day."

Another woman said: "I told my doctor, sorta, but just couldn't get it all out, so he thinks I'm over it. It's too degrading and embarrassing to tell anyone about."

Obviously bulimarexia is much more serious than an extra cookie now and then. These women must learn to be honest and to reach out for support and help in breaking the vicious cycle. This means a willingness to give up their characteristic circular thinking, a way of thought that was well demonstrated by a woman who said, "I want to be helped, but I also want to be skinny. I'd rather be skinny and have this problem than be fat and not have it."

Although bulimarexics are generally slim by any standard, they invariably *feel* fat. They appear to regard their bodies far more critically than so-called normal women or women with other types of emotional problems regard theirs. They are perfectionists. Thin is never thin enough. Their body proportions are *never* right. Their breasts are too small, thighs too big, and so forth.

Laura states: "I'm too heavy chested—34C is not exactly my idea of being comfortable. I feel like a freak."

Sally, who is 4'10" and weighs 110 pounds, says: "I wish my body was petite and tiny. I hate my fat legs! I wish the fat could be wished away."

Jennifer, who is 128 pounds and 5'6", feels "very unattractive if I'm over the weight I desire, even by one pound."

Marie has a petite 5'4" frame that carries all of 108 pounds. She says, "I feel like I'm too heavy now"; and Karen, at 5'8" and 117 reveals, "I love my body when it's thin. I feel hideous and fat when I'm slightly over what feels thin. My self-image is tied up with my physical beauty. I depend on people thinking I'm pretty, and if they don't, I feel crushed."

These subjective comments parallel our clinical impressions and those of many therapists with whom we have worked. In our initial work with bulimarexic college coeds, we were interested in determining the extent of their problems with distorted body image. After a search of the literature, we found a brief, straightforward, instrument, developed by Second and Jourard, called the body cathexis test. Women are asked to rate their feelings about different parts of their body. In order to evaluate the bulimarexic, we added a few questions specifically related to the female self-image (i.e., we elicited their impressions about breasts, thighs, and being a woman). Application of this test to bulimarexic and control subjects in our early research revealed that bulimarexics loathed their bodies to a much greater extent than did women who were suffering from nonfood-related problems. These findings have continued to emerge and suggest that this modified test may be a valuable diagnostic tool in helping to "discover" the elusive, bulimarexic women.

Paradoxically, our data, gleaned from the body cathexis test, also suggest that bulimarexics are quite satisfied with their gender—they very much enjoy being women. These findings cast serious doubt on the traditional "rejection of femininity" hypothesis regarding anorexia/bulimarexia in women.

In addition to feeling revulsion about their own bodies, bulimarexic women are constantly comparing their bodies—and their lives in general—to those of other women—and almost always unfavorably, with further loss of self-esteem. One gymnast who wrote to us expresses this view: "It was inexplicably painful for me just to watch in the gym. I tried to figure out who was better than me, who wasn't so good, who was fatter, and who was thinner. They were doing a complicated exercise while I agonized over the fact that I had just 'pigged out' and I couldn't attempt the movement, even if I wanted to. Feeling absolutely inadequate to do anything about myself, I would run from the gym in tears."

Such striving for perfection only helps to perpetuate feelings of despair and emptiness. On the whole, these women are articulate, bright, and talented, with a potential for creative activity. Many write, paint, dance, or act. However, for most bulimarexics these are activities of the past, activities they once enjoyed but gave up around the time they began to binge. Their conversation is peppered with such phrases as "I used to . . ." or "Once I liked to . . ." In the present, they seem to use their memory of enjoyable activities to *intensify* their problems so that a low-frustration tolerance coupled with unrealistic expectations practically insure failure.

More disturbing, perhaps, is that the lives of bulimarexics are devoid of fun, humor, and genuine self-pleasure. The ability and desire to participate in life joyfully have been left behind; talents and interests that once flourished have been abandoned. Psychologist Eric Berne has said that the road to freedom is through laughter. The ability to laugh also reflects insight into the absurdity of one's irrational beliefs. Humor is often a first therapeutic step toward healing. Bulimarexics, however, are somber and intense. They view life as tragic and hopeless, and their pessimistic philosophy often serves to keep more energetic and positive individuals at a distance. A majority have lost sight of or, in some cases, never discovered the child within—that crazy, fun-loving, exuberant part that permits us to reward ourselves for all we have accomplished. When we lose sight of this, our lives become dreary and meaningless. Bulimarexics typically evidence this loss of perspective.

Recently, we saw a decorative pillow that carried a message relevant to the bulimarexic's distorted sense of self: I MAY NOT BE TO-TALLY PERFECT, BUT PARTS OF ME ARE EXCELLENT. Unfortunately, this concept is foreign to the bulimarexic who has an "ideal weight" in mind. This magic figure is definitely on the thin side but is not clinically unhealthy as in anorexia. Those who force vomit seem to have an easier time maintaining their ideal weight than those who offset binges by fasting and dieting over longer periods of time. They weigh themselves so frequently that they can detect minute changes and act on them immediately. On the other hand, weight fluctuations in women who fast and diet after bingeing are typically more dramatic, often ranging from twenty to twenty-five pounds. One thirty-six-year-old woman writes: "I binge three or four months at a time and have since junior high school. I eat everything in sight. During my binges, my weight goes up to 150 or 180. My best weight is 115 and I'm 5′6″ tall. Now I'm in my 'fat phase,' and I'm a physical wreck. I feel tired and unsocial. I dread being seen!"

Another woman discusses her severe cycles of weight gain/weight loss: "I've been living with this syndrome for five years. I am now twenty years old. My life is a perpetual diet, along with insatiable binges! I've lost one hundred pounds in eighteen months. I've had many relationships and when they end I inevitably feast."

It is often difficult if not impossible to relegate women to one diagnostic category or another. Some bulimarexic women would be classified as obese during their "fat" phases. In addition, 10 to 12 percent of the bulimarexic women we have treated report having been diagnosed as anorexic earlier in their lives. Several were hospitalized in order to bring their weight to medically acceptable levels. Furthermore, recent studies of women's attitudes toward food indicate that more and more so-called normal women are evidencing anorexiclike symptoms. This suggests that women without personality abnormalities are being pressured by unrealistic cultural standards regarding slimness. Many seem to be adopting behavior patterns quite similar to those of anorexic and bulimarexic women.

In bulimarexia one behavior elicits and sustains another. The "bulimarexic motto" might be: I eat to purge and I purge to eat. The disorder rarely begins as a full-blown cycle. In fact, most bulimarexics go through a phase where they are dieting and perhaps vomiting occasionally, but they are still in control. In other words, the binge and purge episodes represent interruptions in an otherwise normal life. This early stage is short-lived and seems to end primarily because the women believe they have discovered the miracle of weight control through purging. In an overwhelming number of women, this destructive insight occurred during adolescence or early adulthood. The following two comments are typical:

My earliest memories of the bingeing pattern that was to be with me for the next twelve years began in adolescence. At about the age of fourteen, my best friend and I began to center our lives around visits to the neighborhood store for food, devouring packaged cakes and chocolate sundaes! If we had no money, anything we could find in her refrigerator would do. Needless to say, I began to gain weight and became quite chubby. At the end of tenth grade, I decided to lose ten pounds in order to become a cheerleader. That was the year I had my first boyfriend and was ecstatic. I was relying heavily on fasting to stay slim, which I found unbearable. In school we read about the Roman vomitoriums and I was intrigued. At first, I didn't employ this wondrous method very often but soon I reached the point where no matter what I put into my stomach, I had my fingers down my throat shortly thereafter.

I began bingeing and starving at age fifteen after losing fifteen pounds on a diet. This went on for a year after I became tired of starving, and I gained thirty pounds. Having no success with dieting because I wouldn't stick to it, I began to take laxatives on occasion (one to three times per week). I then began to binge and vomit, which has been going on daily for the last two and a half years.

Forced vomiting is the most dramatic and immediate method of purging. It also appears to be the most common, perhaps because it seems to be the easiest and most efficient form of weight control. Needless to say, it may also be the most self-destructive. The issue of immediacy is probably central because women often say that they can throw up before the calories have a chance to take effect. Vomiting also provides instant relief for their painfully overstuffed bellies.

Bulimarexics often refer to "learning" to throw up. In other words, they learn about it as a method of controlling weight. In the beginning, they seem to think it is a great new discovery. The following story illustrates this:

"In my sophomore year of high school, I learned to put my fingers down my throat to make myself throw up. I had stopped eating normal meals and would very often fast for days at a time. That Thanksgiving I had just eaten too much, and I felt I was going to be sick. I was in the bathroom with my sister and cousin, and one of them said, 'Well, if it's going to come up, why don't you stick your fingers down your throat and help it up.' No sooner said than done. I felt thin again immediately and thought, 'This is great! I just ate the most delicious, fattening dinner and I won't gain any weight.' "

The length of a binge depends primarily upon the method of purging. For those who purge via fasting, the entire binge/purge cycle may last a few days or extend to several months. One woman binged every day or so, then gave up eating altogether for at least twenty-four hours, sometimes forty-eight. Another had a cycle of bingeing for one day, then dieting strenuously for the next few days. This meant skipping breakfast, having plain yogurt for lunch, and eating hard-boiled eggs and a vegetable for dinner. ("I chew gum when I feel like snacking. If I want to lose weight quickly, I limit myself to two hard-boiled eggs a day.") Still another, after periods of bingeing, would go on a series of drastic diets, the most serious of which was a "meat" diet. "All that I ate for eleven weeks was six ounces of meat a day and diet soda; I lost thirty-five pounds and gained it back in two months, for I immediately began bingeing again." For those who purge by forced vomiting or laxative abuse, the cycle is generally complete within an hour or two.

Other women learn about purging methods from friends. The technique was introduced to another adolescent by a veteran camper at a camp for overweight young adults; this person put it quite literally when she commented, "I found it a great way to have my cake and eat it, too." Still another read an article about gymnasts that mentioned the method. And there is Nicole, whose boyfriend jokingly suggested that she vomit after she complained one night about "pigging out."

Bulimarexics are suggestible women. It is unfortunate that a chance remark from family or even from a physician (one woman heard a doctor talk about "skinny girls who threw up") can lead to a syndrome that approaches addiction. The fact that bulimarexia is rampant in this country, especially on college campuses, has led some people to wonder whether or not it is contagious, in the manner of a disease. As we point out several times in this book, the *syndrome itself* is not contagious. It is a learned behavior. What is contagious is the passing along of the purge and the reliance upon it as a magic solution to weight control.

In addition to forced vomiting, other methods of purging are commonly utilized. Laxative abuse is quite frequent, as are diuretic and emetic abuse, fasting, and enemas. The women are likely to exercise compulsively, swimming many laps, running many miles, working out with weights. Some women combine different methods of exercise as well as experimenting with bizarre diets. A small percentage of women we have treated spend hours chewing food and spitting it out.

In order to facilitate vomiting, many bulimarexics rely on Q-tips and similar initiators because they prove more effective and less "disgusting" than fingers. They soon learn that drinking copious amounts of fluids facilitates vomiting. Some maintain that certain foods, such as chocolate, are useful in initiating diarrhea. As time goes by, with practice, most of them find that vomiting occurs spontaneously each time they eat. By this time, of course, their bodies have suffered grievously, and medical attention is necessary.

The actual length of time women spend bingeing and purging can be misleading and irrelevant. They spend far more time in obsessive rumination about food, either attempting to stave off a binge or actually preparing for one. Many of these women appear to love to cook, which leads relatives and friends to overlook other aspects of their obsession. "I collect recipes," one woman wrote us. "I've sent away for every recipe booklet I could find, and my prized possessions are booklets with pictures of gooey, rich desserts. I especially like to torture myself by looking at these pictures while dieting, and I make lists of all the foods I'll eat when my diet is over. I tell my family and friends, several times a day, about the pizza I'm going to have when I get off this diet."

Other women enjoy planning elaborate dinners or large cocktail parties with "fifty different types of hors d'oeuvres." They constantly pore over cookbooks and are often praised as excellent hostesses. When the obsession with food leads to hoarding—as it frequently does—the torture becomes even more exquisite and the anxiety that results is extreme: "I feel obligated to eat what I've already hoarded because I don't want to waste what I've bought." Another woman admitted: "I feel extremely nervous when I've hoarded so much food that I no longer have a place to hide it. When I have guests, I lock all cabinets, and if they should look into the refrigerator, I tell them a neighbor's fridge is being repaired and she's keeping all the food in mine."

Bulimarexics typically binge on high-calorie junk foods, the kind of food that may have been forbidden in childhood. Their selection of food may reflect defiance. Flavor and taste do not seem to be important, with sweets and fried foods, such as french fries, predominating. As time goes on, most become less and less discriminating about what they eat. "The foods are uglier and uglier, like globs of fried flour, oil, and sugar." Caloric intake per binge can range from one thousand to twenty thousand calories.

Obviously the single most important precondition to bingeing is being alone (although some women do report having a few cronies engaged in the same behavior). If the bulimarexic can count on being alone at night, she is more apt to binge at night. However, women caught up in this cycle are ingenious at finding places and times when they can be alone—at home, at work, and even in restaurants. At college, they may eat normal meals with roommates in communal dining places but still find ways to slip food to their rooms afterward: "I think I'll get more pleasure out of it in my room. If I hear someone coming, I hide the food." Many women admit that if they were constantly supervised, they probably would not binge.

It is not surprising that bulimarexics have few friends—so much of their time is spent in supporting their habit and in keeping others from knowing about it. Some refuse to answer the telephone or the doorbell while under the influence of their "fat attacks." Others are simply too worn out from bingeing to accept invitations or are afraid they will not be able to keep the date when the time comes. "If I was bingeing and someone knocked on my door, I wouldn't answer. I'd tell people I'd be there and never show up."

The following insightful statement sums it up: "Friends, that was a major problem. I knew a lot of people, but was alienating them because I couldn't be around them with the cycle I was in. There were all those people who were there for me to do things with if I was willing to say, 'Hey, do you want to come over?' I was scared to do it . . . to develop close friends."

A few bulimarexic women are drawn into relationships with other lonely and unhappy women. This often serves to reinforce their weaknesses rather than enhance their strengths. Jan would binge with a friend at college: "I can remember one night, a low point in my life . . . we found every nickel we could and ran to the candy machine. There was only one kind of candy left, a peanut bar which we both disliked. Yet we pumped coins into that machine, on full stomachs, eating one peanut bar after another while crying, 'Why are we doing this?' "

Despite the enormous amount of time and energy expended in bingeing and purging, many bulimarexic women manage to maintain high academic averages in college. By their own admission, they are overachievers. They tend to compensate for their perceived shortcomings by driving themselves, and when their talents are recognized they both thrive on and dislike the recognition ("I needed it to justify my awfulness and hated it because I felt undeserving"). However, the drive for academic success is often related to pleasing others and to the expectation of "marrying well" rather than to the personal joy of intellectual achievement. The expectation is that such achievement will lead to the fulfillments that marriage and childbearing can bring. For example, a doctor is more likely to meet and be attracted to a woman who is well educated; a woman is most likely to meet "her man" in a college or university. So achievement is seen mainly in terms of what rewards it can elicit from others, particularly men.

Most of these women describe themselves as never having had an intimate relationship with a man. Given their behavior, intimacy is difficult if not impossible. Many continue to believe that social failure is due to their appearance and try to avoid dating altogether. Others become supremely critical of the men they encounter or adopt a clinging, possessive style with men who typically reject or otherwise abuse them. Even so, relationships with men are considered primary, and friendships with women, when they do exist, are often terminated when a man enters the picture. At best, relationships with women are likely to be superficial since the bulimarexic is in constant competition with other women. She runs the risk of losing out on both counts.

This basically dishonest lifestyle often leads to more deviant behaviors. Not surprisingly, bulimarexics become adept at lying. Stealing is also frequent. They steal food from roommates ("I don't care if she's my best friend!"), family, and from stores and supermarkets. Some also steal money in order to restore depleted food supplies. Several women told us of having been arrested for shoplifting food. Confrontations with roommates or relatives over missing food supplies can lead to rifts and the kind of isolation that is the last thing the bulimarexic needs. One woman's story provides an example: "Sneaking food was always a great treat. I got to eat the food (first bonus) and nobody knew about it (second bonus). As an annual ritual my aunt baked Christmas pies several weeks before the holiday, and then froze them so we couldn't eat them beforehand. I snuck down to the freezer and ate them frozen! Unfortunately, I was caught and haven't been invited back."

Added to the bulimarexic's feelings of anxiety and shame is the sheer necessity of paying for the huge amounts of food consumed. Few women can afford the financial outlay. For those who are married or living with families, this means outright stealing of money or ingenious camouflage of food bills (in addition to hiding evidence of bingeing). It would not be an exaggeration to say that the cost of food for the bulimarexic could equal a large family's average food bill. Nicole, whose story began this chapter, would visit different stores each day so that replacement of food eaten in a binge would not be noticed. Another woman spent as much time devising ways of hiding food bills from her husband as she did bingeing and purging. Major charge cards proved useful because she could then make purchases at specialty stores in addition to grocery stores and supermarkets; the bills from each grocery store seemed smaller. For Nicole and other women like her, guilt becomes a constant companion (Nicole was literally "vomiting all the food my boyfriend and family worked so hard to buy"). And, sadly, energy that could be directed toward positive endeavors is dissipated in attempting to hide the bulimarexic behavior.

Some natural questions arise: What do these women get out of bingeing and purging? What are the consequences? Are there rewards, payoffs? Ironically, it seems that there *are* for the bulimarexic, at least for the short term. Some describe bingeing as a marvelous, albeit transient, release. This frenzied high inevitably leads to a more relaxed state; once they begin to binge, they report feeling calm. Since many bulimarexics report troubled sleep patterns and insomnia, they frequently use bingeing as a kind of sleeping pill. Others describe the ecstasy of relinquishing control and surrendering to food. Some admit that their bizarre behavior makes them feel unique, gives them a feeling of specialness.

Purging then becomes a purification rite, a means of overcoming self-loathing by gaining self-control. Having reestablished their disciplined ways, the bulimarexics feel "good" and perceive themselves as the perfect human beings they strive to be. In describing the purge or the process of getting ready for the purge, some say they feel "completely fresh, clean again." A phrase often heard is "a new beginning." However, their feelings of self-worth are only temporary, and the fear persists that the binge compulsion will overwhelm them once again. It nearly always does. Since these women are convinced that they are unlovable and inadequate, they are extremely sensitive to even minor slights and frustrations, which will soon be used as an excuse to initiate another binge.

Rejection, confrontation, disappointments, and anxiety are often major precursors of a binge. The decision to binge, more often than not, is related to the inability of bulimarexic women to assert themselves and deal with their problems in a direct way. Anger is a rare emotion for these women; they have been well socialized to be agreeable, compliant, and nonassertive. Their immediate response to disappointment and pain is to feel hopeless and helpless rather than angry. Most lack awareness of their inability to express anger and rationalize their need for control in a number of ways, i.e., "If I get angry, I will go completely crazy"; "If I allow myself to get angry and speak up, it will hurt other people"; "If I acknowledge my own human rights to be honest and angry, I will turn people off and be rejected." This sense of shame and guilt over their disordered eating pattern also effectively helps them to suppress anger. Thus, the action and problem solving that can follow the experience of anger and assertion—the very things that can result in productive change—are denied to most bulimarexics. They are stuck with the tried and true "feminine" way of dealing with pain and discomfort.

Bulimarexics report gorging and purging for some of the following reasons:

- As a way of avoiding failure. A woman may be anxious about writing a college term paper or making a difficult phone call. She may binge instead of taking action or may postpone taking responsibility by first bingeing and then tackling the assignment that causes her anxiety. The student who flunks her exam may remark that she failed because she binged the night before rather than admitting that she failed because she did not prepare for the exam.

- As a way of handling the stress involved in new activities, particularly social encounters. The bulimarexic's pattern of obsessional thinking allows her to separate from the person or people she is with at the moment. One woman expressed it this way: "I attended a party that included some well-known people. As usual, I felt tongue-tied, dumb, and inconsequential. As usual, I smiled sweetly and engaged in chitchat. All the time I was secretly planning a midnight binge when I returned home." Another says: "I began bingeing in order to alleviate the anxieties I had about undertaking new things and to provide myself with an excuse to take a rest from everything once in a while."

- As a way of postponing sexual relations, as graphically expressed by the statement, "I'm too stuffed to want sex," or as a way of loving oneself when a sexual encounter is disappointing. The following statement is illustrative: "I say to myself, 'I love you (meaning me), even if *he* doesn't, so go ahead and *eat* if it makes you feel loved.' "

- As a way of eliciting attention and getting back at those people who the bulimarexic feels *made* her binge in the first place. This is, of course, the ultimate way of avoiding responsibility for the behavior.

The resolution to stop bingeing forever is an important part of the cycle since it guarantees failure. Bulimarexics typically believe that total abstinence from forbidden foods is the only acceptable way of gaining control. Some are able to give up bingeing for a considerable time—up to three or four months if their lives are running smoothly—but a rejection or even a minor disappointment can trigger a binge. Instead of congratulating themselves for what they have accomplished and acknowledging that they have made *one* mistake, they use the binge as an excuse for continuing as before. Having succumbed to one cookie or one piece of chocolate cream pie, they consider themselves out of control. The old "dieter's guilt," as one woman put it, takes over: "Since I've already blown it, why stop?"

Feeling themselves powerless in the moment, victims of near mystical forces that propel them toward uncontrolled eating, many women use a variety of techniques to aid themselves in their attempts to stave off bingeing. They make endless lists of chores to keep themselves busy every minute of the day, keep journals, and write down complicated rules to which they must adhere. Some write inspirational notes to themselves, outlining resolutions and responsibilities. Others move from one strenuous diet to another. Still others literally move to a new apartment or job when the behavior becomes extreme. Thus, they delude themselves that they are "fighting" the behavior. Their days, which typically begin with good intentions and lists of things to do, usually deteriorate from control to chaos.

In time, the bingeing and purging become habitual, and precipitating factors become irrelevant because bingeing then occurs at any time and under any circumstance—when these women are happy, sad, excited, under stress, or depressed. The pattern has become an entrenched and crippling coping mechanism that is a major part of the bulimarexic's lifestyle.

The dilemma that results is well expressed by this woman: "It's easy to sit over an open half gallon of ice cream and find solace in that—but it certainly is nowhere near living."

3.

Socialization and the Family

MONTH after month we sit in a room with a group of very special women. They have vitality, talent, wit, and energy. The fact that they are also generally slim and attractive is quite secondary. What is primary—and tragic—is their inability to acknowledge their particular assets and their uniqueness. They are like championship thoroughbreds that wear blinders and run on circular tracks. Unlike thoroughbreds, however, they do not try to outrun their trackmates. Bulimarexics not only run on circular tracks with blinders, they also are too preoccupied with themselves to think about winning the race. In fact, they usually expect to lose! And as we have seen, these women of high potential feel that the only way they can win is by being thin, thin enough to attain an ideal that might, just possibly, be unattainable. What has made them this way? What pressures make the women we treat feel that they should be paper dolls, all cut to one pattern?

Researchers and feminists have had much to say about these matters and have come up with a number of interesting conclusions, many of them centering around the socialization of women. While it is not possible for us to cover all these theories in this book, we do want to touch upon those that seem relevant to the women we are treating.

Until recently, it was thought that a woman could be fulfilled only as wife and mother. Whatever energies were left over could be devoted to volunteer activities or personal hobbies (generally undertaken without pay and in "spare time"). Women who sought to achieve in other areas were considered to be making adjustments that were substitutes for the feminine role. There were exceptions, of course. For reasons that have nothing to do with personal fulfillment, many women have had to work in order to augment family income. Others have gone against the grain of what was considered acceptable to pursue their own goals. But the tendency has been to view these women with a degree of alarm. The main goal for a woman was to appeal to and catch a man. After that, protected economically (and perhaps emotionally), the roles of wife and mother would involve her totally. The traditional boast of her husband was, "My wife doesn't work," and she subscribed to this notion as well.

As Susie Orbach pointed out in *Fat Is a Feminist Issue,* "To get a man, a woman has to learn to regard herself as an item, a commodity, a sex object. Much of her experience and identity depends on how she and others see her." She attempts to conform to what "others will find pleasing and attractive" and also to what she *perceives* them to consider pleasing and attractive. The ideal woman, as presented in newspaper advertisements, in magazines, and on television—whether in commercials or in the programs themselves—becomes the ideal to which she should ascribe. Orbach goes on to point out how women are made to believe that "the body is not satisfactory as it is." The woman must deodorize and perfume it, bind it up or let it hang free, and scramble to renew the clothes that quickly become out-of-date according to the vagaries of fashion.

The feminine ideal itself has not remained constant throughout the ages. At times slimness has been prized, and at other times a certain degree of plumpness has received admiration. During some eras—the Victorian period, for instance—a modified version of *both* body types was desired simultaneously. Women of this time are pictured with ample hips and bosoms but with painfully constricted tiny waists. But no matter what the historical period, the common denominator for women has likely been the urge to conform.

In our own time, the exhortation has been for women to be

thin. Certainly the fashion models in advertisements of forty years ago seem well cushioned in comparison with those to whom we are accustomed today. A careful perusal of the ads over the years will show us that models are becoming more and more emaciated, until an ideal that approaches anorexia exists.

Some researchers feel that extreme slimness is valued in industrial societies where food is plenteous. Others maintain that body ideal is related to the degree of freedom women enjoy in a particular era. For instance, Kim Chernin, in her book *The Obsession: Reflections on the Tyranny of Slenderness,* postulates that during periods of history when women are tied into their mothering and nurturing roles and are without personal power, they are "allowed" to appear more female, with emphasis on distinctive female characteristics (full breasts and hips). Conversely, in times when women are more liberated, the ideal of slimness, even boyishness, is in vogue. This could be seen in the twenties, when women joined the burst of freedom after World War I, and within the last several decades when women made their way into the workplace in increasing numbers.

Along with the current pursuit of slimness, there has been a similar obsession with youth. Once mothers and daughters were distinguished from each other very clearly by their clothing. A mother's clothing reflected her maturity—or at least the maturity of her years. But fashions for both groups have become virtually indistinguishable, and it is not at all unusual for mothers and daughters to exchange clothes with each other. As Bess Myerson, once Miss America and now involved with public service, commented when this phenomenon took hold: "We used to dress like Jackie Kennedy, now we're dressing like Caroline."

The cults of slimness and of youthfulness were perhaps best personified by a young British model who first appeared on the American scene in 1966. Nicknamed Twiggy, and she did indeed resemble a twig, Lesley Hornby Armstrong was seventeen-years-old and at 5'7" weighed ninety-seven pounds. Her hair was cropped, and her eyes, heavily made-up, gave her the appearance of waifishness. Soon her body, with its 31-22-32 measurements, caused a furor when it was featured in fashion magazine advertisements, and countless numbers of American women began to pattern their clothes styles, makeup, hairstyles—and finally their bodies—after hers.

Later, Hilde Bruch, in *Eating Disorders: Obesity, Anorexia Nervosa and the Person Within,* and a number of other experts in the field of eating disorders pointed an accusing finger at Twiggy and felt there was a correlation between her arrival in the United States and the appalling increase of diagnosed cases of anorexia nervosa. (The binge/purge syndrome as an eating disorder was still in the closet at that time.) Researcher Ann Beuf of the University of Pennsylvania reminded us that the first outbreak of these disorders occurred directly after World War I, when the flapper type of woman was in style. One wonders if a person like Twiggy, singlehandedly as it were, could have established the trend in body type that has become so relentlessly pursued in recent years. Undoubtedly, the situation is more complex than that. However, Twiggy made her American debut at a time when the youth of America were a large and potent group of consumers. The baby boom infants, born after World War II, were adolescents, with their own money and their own power. Their numbers were legion, and their heroes were the mop-haired Beatles, the four young men from England who captured the American music scene and who looked like exuberant little boys.

So it might be said that young was in and slim was in, and big business hastened to cash in on both trends. The fashion industry formed and re-formed the ideal image (with variations on the same theme). During the unisex decade of the sixties, girls tended to look like boys and boys looked like girls—or, more accurately, both looked like little boys. Then for both sexes the long, thick bangs of the Beatles gave way to flowing locks. From the rear, it was often impossible to determine a young person's identity. And if the trend to wear trousers for all occasions seemed to imply freedom for women, there were certain aspects of fashion that continued to hamper them. In her book *The Language of Clothes,* Alison Lurie notes the footgear for women wearing pants: stiletto heels, clogs, platform shoes. Throughout the book, Lurie assesses the history of female fashion as a "series of more or less successful campaigns to force, flatter or bribe women back into uncomfortable and awkward styles, not only for the purpose of vicarious ostentation and security of sexual ownership, but also and increasingly in order to handicap them in professional competition with men."

Another phenomenon appeared after the advent of Twiggy. The diet industry burgeoned into big business, catering to the national pursuit of slimness. Today, as we all know, it is impossible to turn on the television or to riffle through a magazine without having the "slim" message hammered at us. In spring diet articles appear like flowers, urging us to anticipate bathing suit season. Even our social conversations invariably turn to diet groups, diet books, or the pros and cons of new diets that are currently being promoted. All of this has fed into—and continues to feed into—the consciousness of young women, who believe that if they can conform to the ideal, be perfect in body, life's major problems will magically be solved.

Now let us examine some of the other aspects that enter into the socialization of women. It might be useful to run through a brief history of the mothers, and sometimes the grandmothers, of the young women we are treating for eating disorders today. For these young women are the daughters of the first generation of women to have attended Weight Watchers. We will take a look at fathers as well.

During World War II, for reasons of patriotism and for money, millions of women (Rosie the Riveter) joined the labor force or various branches of the armed forces. When the war was over, it was assumed that most of them would relinquish their jobs in favor of returning veterans. The veterans themselves, with savings in hand and eligible for Veterans Administration and Federal Housing Administration benefits, were eager to own their own homes. Newly married to young women, some of whom were graduating from college in the forties and early fifties, they began the exodus to the suburbs. The nuclear family as we know it today became the American dream, with the husband/father who commuted to work in the city, the stay-at-home mother who tended the household and children, and the children who would receive all the benefits of fresh air and space and the privilege of growing up in a nonindustrial community.

Family life revolved around one father, one mother, and their children, with each family unit ensconced in a house that might be identical with or similar to other houses on the suburban scene. As generally happens after wartime, there was a trend toward larger families. With little or no household help and lacking the support of female relatives who might once have lent a hand with child rearing, young mothers—even those whose hopes for personal achievement might have been raised through college education—found it necessary to set aside individual concerns. Wives became chauffeurs for children and also for husbands who typically returned from the city at night or, in extreme cases, only on weekends. Feeling alone and isolated, yet indebted to their husbands for the economic security that made the dream of the suburbs reality, these women submerged themselves in the roles of wife and mother.

At first many were ecstatic, as Betty Friedan recalls in her book *It Changed My Life: Writings on the Women's Movement:* "I felt that I would never again, ever, be so happy as I was living in Queens. The floors were parquet, and the ceilings were molded white plaster, no pipes, and the plumbing worked. . . . And now our friends were the other couples like us, with kids at the nursery school who squealed at each other. . . . It was fun at first, shopping in those new supermarkets. And we bought barbecue grills, and made dips out of sour cream and dried onion soup to serve with potato chips, while our husbands made the martinis as dry as in the city and cooked hamburgers on the charcoal, and we sat in canvas chairs on our terrace and thought how beautiful our children looked, playing in the twilight, and how lucky we all were, and that it would last forever."

The media and big business had an investment in keeping women in the kitchen, at home, and in the role of consumers, and wondrous new appliances were manufactured for their benefit—

washers, dryers, and refrigerators in decorator colors. The American housewife as the centerpiece in her gleaming kitchen was glorified. As Betty Friedan reminds us: in *It Changed My Life* "It certainly didn't occur to any of us then, even the most radical, that companies which made a big profit selling us all those washing machines, dryers, freezers, and second cars were overselling us on the bliss of domesticity in order to sell us more things. Even the most radical of us, in our innocence, wanted those pressure cookers." The woman involved with children, taking care of a home and a man, was made to feel essential: "At home, you were necessary, you were important, you were the boss, in fact—the mother— and the new mystique gave it the rationale of career."

The feminine mystique, glorifying woman as mother and homemaker, served to keep her complacent, satisfied, and "lucky to have what she had." The small world of the kitchen, nursery, and bedroom reinforced woman's traditional role as the caretaker who needed to be taken care of.

However, as the decade of the fifties moved on, the picture changed. Many women began to wonder whether their suburban dream houses were prisons. Feelings of boredom, confusion, and meaninglessness emerged. When these women presented their "symptoms" to doctors, they were often given pills—to pep them up or calm them down—and told to buy a new dress or to devise new ways of satisfying their husbands and of gaining rewards from the mother/wife role. Experts advised the women to "escape" from the home for an occasional outing, failing to realize the extent of the problem. Many vulnerable women found the outings and pills insufficient. Midafternoon drinking provided relief, a phenomenon that increased to the point where sociologist Jessie Bernard concluded in *The Future of Marriage* that "the housewife syndrome might well be viewed as public health problem number one."

In 1957 Betty Friedan sent an intensive questionnaire to her college classmates, fifteen years after their graduation from Smith. Alarmingly, her classmates, the majority of whom were middle-class housewives and mothers, described their lives as "incomplete" and "empty" and themselves as "almost nonexistent." At the age of forty, they were questioning the meaning of their lives and regretting their decisions to give up or forego careers for marriage.

By 1963 Friedan had expanded her findings into a book she called *The Feminine Mystique,* and "the problem that has no name burst like a boil through the image of the happy American Housewife." It is difficult for young women of today to fully comprehend the confusion, excitement, and pain this book generated, as women realized that the problem that had no name was their problem too. Marlene was one of these women. Having completed her undergraduate work at the University of North Carolina, she had abandoned her dream of graduate school when her then husband decided to relocate in order to continue work on his Ph.D. Without questioning how it would affect her life, Marlene agreed to the move and to the need to help him complete his graduate training. This meant working as a salesperson in a department store, the only job available to a woman with a B.A. in fine arts in the city to which they moved. Twin daughters were born to her in 1963, followed by a son in 1965. Shortly after the birth of her son, as she cared for three children under three, Marlene read *The Feminine Mystique,* two years after its publication. Through tears, she realized that she was not alone. With relief, she discovered that the anger, helplessness, and hopelessness that she was experiencing were shared by thousands of other women.

The Feminine Mystique galvanized women as it hit them where they were weakest, in the depths of their unawareness and passivity. In exploding the myth that all a woman needed to be happy was wifehood and motherhood, Friedan awakened a new wave of feminism that has helped to change society in important ways. She urged women to develop their own potential, to return to college and careers, and to fulfill themselves in meaningful work. At the time, this was a large order. Educational and career opportunities, particularly in the professions, were still denied to women. Discrimination against women worked in subtle ways, both in occupational settings and in universities. Financial aid, more often than not, was forthcoming for "putting the husband" through his education, but married women found themselves unable to compete for federal scholarships and loan aid because of the difficulty of managing both schooling and the home front. There were, of course, many other women who had never developed skills or whose skills had become rusty during the years of homemaking. For these women, the frustration intensified. Although aware of the problem, they felt there was no place to go.

In the late sixties, the number of American women who were being psychiatrically "serviced" began to increase measurably. Pauline Bart, a sociologist at the University of Illinois, studied a large group of middle-class women who were patients in psychiatric hospitals. Suffering from what came to be called the "Empty Nest Syndrome," these women had become depressed when their children left home and were eventually institutionalized. Younger women with agoraphobia (the fear of being alone in a large open space) formed another distinct group in need of psychiatric help. As increased educational and occupational opportunities opened up, women with the aspiration but not the skills to cope with the responsibilities involved began to suffer from performance anxiety (a neurosis that had been thought to lie primarily in the realm of male psychiatric dysfunction).

Unfortunately, therapy often served to increase the women's sense of powerlessness and became an effective tool in further controlling them. There were few women therapists, and of those that there were, only a handful embraced a feminist orientation. Female patients, accustomed to male authority, preferred men therapists. Phyllis Chesler emphasizes this point in *Women and Madness:* "In 1960, the membership of the American Psychiatric Association totaled 11,083 of whom 10,000 were men and 1,083 were women. In 1970, their membership increased to 17,298 of whom 14,267 were men and 3,031 were women. Thus, 90 percent of all psychiatrists during the 1960s were men." In addition, many therapists, both psychologists and psychiatrists, were still rooted in psychoanalytic theory and accepted, lived out, and practiced stereotypical attitudes toward women in their own lives. Instead of directly addressing their patients' present and critical problems, therapists often redirected women's energy to the past and to intellectualizing rather than doing, acting, changing and growing in the present. Therapy was deemed successful when the "woman came to her senses" and got married or became pregnant. More often than not, therapy reinforced acceptance of the traditional female role.

This message, then, was transmitted to the daughters of these women. By and large, middle-class parents of the fifties were upwardly mobile, eager to provide their children with the material and intellectual advantages they may have felt they were denied. Often this meant a college education. However, expectations for male and female children were different. For young men, a college education was the ticket to career success and financial security. For women, the expected reward was marriage to a potentially successful, well-educated man, and it was important for women to "keep up" with their husbands. While young women might be praised for academic achievement during college, as the undergraduate years drew to a close, pressures increased to propel them toward popularity with the opposite sex and, eventually, an appropriate marriage. Well-intentioned parents wanted their daughters to be well taken care of, and the daughters themselves were eager for family approval.

In sum, as sociologist Lenore Weitzman points out in a chapter in *Women: A Feminist Perspective:* "The well-socialized American girl learns three clear lessons: one concerning her personality, a second concerning her capability, and a third concerning her future role. With regard to her personality, she 'knows' that to be truly feminine she will be sweet, expressive, not too intelligent, nurturing, cooperative, pretty, and fairly passive. With regard to her capability, she 'knows' she will always be less capable and less important than most men. With regard to her future, she 'knows' she will be a wife and mother. If she is a successful women, she will acquire this status soon. . . ."

During the sixties, the culture as a whole was experiencing a number of changes that caused upheavals in traditional attitudes and behavior. The Civil Rights movement attracted thousands of middle-class students and provided them with shocking revelations about life beyond their secure suburban communities. Other teenagers and students began to repudiate the materialism and "false" values of their parents and joined protests for an end to American involvement in Vietnam and for greater student control of education and free speech on campuses. Another contingent of young people broke away from their families to drop out as hippies, runaways, and flower children.

In addition to these revolutionary changes, the advent of oral contraceptives led to a "sexual revolution." With the fear of pregnancy virtually eliminated by the pill, women were encouraged toward a sexual openness that was once thought primarily the province of men. Young women might have intercourse with the men whom they expected to marry, but premarital sex with a number of partners had not been the general rule. Now there was pressure to be freer, not to be "uptight and guilty," and for many women the so-called sexual revolution led to a new kind of anxiety. Multiple sexual contacts might give a temporary illusion of desirability, but women now experienced sex in ways that removed it from the realm of intimacy, security, and a feeling of connectedness. Beneath the freedom lay the conditioning to dependency that had characterized women, and the desire for a permanent connection remained. The lack of boundaries in relationships with the opposite sex often created new fears because suddenly nothing was predictable, and the comfort of familiar rules (and roles) appeared no longer to be there. This existential desperation drove many women to compete with each other more than ever for the attention of men, thus creating a self-consciousness about physical attractiveness and youth that was particularly intense. Here, again, advertisers and manufacturers found easy prey among these women preoccupied with being slim and young.

The decade of the seventies brought continued change for women. The burgeoning feminist movement resulted in women's consciousness raising groups and in a desire among women for increasing control over their bodies and their lives in general. New career opportunities opened up, and women were encouraged to express themselves with more assertion. But the pressures to succeed, along with heightened insecurity from unstable relationships, competition at work, and the increased incidence of divorce, took their toll. A number of studies conducted in the seventies indicated that under the cloak of feminism, the entrenched feminine modes of response remained. In many ways, women were talking like feminists, but continuing to act out the conventionally feminine fantasies and roles.

Barbara Ehrenreich and Deirdre English (in their book *For Her Own Good: 150 Years of the Experts' Advice to Women*) show that the slogan "You've come a long way, baby" was debatable. In pointing out that the seventies produced an ambiguous and frustrating form of liberation, they say: "After the old dependency came the new insecurity of shifting relationships, a competitive work world, unstable marriages—an insecurity from which no woman could count herself 'safe' and settled. There was a sense of being adrift, but now there was no one to turn to. . . ." Socialization had conditioned many women to be dependent, passive, and noncompetitive, and they were unprepared for new roles.

IN the decade of the eighties, researchers began to find a profound sex-role conflict in eating-disorder subjects. Anorexics in one study scored lower on the masculinity scale of the *Bem Sex Role Inventory* (BSRI) than normal controls. The researchers hypothesized that these women had failed to develop certain traditionally "masculine" assertive and independent traits that may be essential in our present society. Further studies found that a group of bulimarexics scored lower than normal women on *all* sex-typed items of the BSRI. These results seemed to indicate low self-esteem and a poorly defined sense of self among these women. Researchers at the Carrier Foundation hypothesized that associated psychopathology, particularly depression, might account for such findings. They, therefore, compared the sex-role self-perceptions of their eating-disorder patients with those of depressed female psychiatric patients with no history of eating disorder. Their study also extended the examination of sex-role self-perceptions to *ideal* self-perceptions. They found lower masculine self-ratings in eating-disorder patients, as had been previously reported but found that depression, not eating disturbance, was responsible for the lower masculine self-ratings on the *Bem Inventory*. In addition, their eating-disorder patients described their *ideal* selves as significantly more "feminine." These findings reinforced our own view that bulimarexia is directly related to overcompliance with society's perception of femininity.

Regarding this point we have our own observation. The climate has changed, and it is no longer fashionable for women to admit that they embrace traditional feminine values. However, what we feel and what we do is often quite different. Conflicting messages beset women from all sides. The question "What does it mean to be a woman?" often elicits nervous laughter from college audiences. No matter how strong and sophisticated a woman may be in activities related to career, there are always areas in which she feels powerless.

Recently we watched a television program that poignantly expressed the no-win alternatives for many contemporary women. A group of foreign correspondents were being interviewed by a well-known talk-show personality. Intelligent, courageous, and sensitive, these women were all single and in their twenties and thirties. Without exception, they loved their work. It had been a long haul getting there. They felt special, fortunate, and grateful. Their climb to the top had been hard, and they had encountered resistance. The final few minutes of the show were particularly revealing. In spite of their love of their work, these women longed for children, husbands, and homes. At the same time, they were afraid that men could not tolerate the rigors of a correspondent's life, and they agonized over the effects their work might have on children.

Experts in eating disorders who observe these conflicts in their clients often encourage traditional feminine values and discourage masculine strivings in a manner that is reminiscent of "anatomy is destiny." They believe excessive dieting expresses a rejection of femininity, an inability to cope with the demands of adult womanhood. Thus, masculine strivings are deviant, and by extension the feminist movement is criticized as being responsible for the dramatic increase in eating disorders. William Davis, director of the Center for the Study of Anorexia and Bulimia, expresses this view: "Contemporary women are inundated with the image of the 'liberated female,' someone who is defined as aggressive, assertive and ambitious. Traditionally, these characteristics have been a part of the male role, and it is only recently that women have been exhorted to conquer, overcome and master. As a result, adolescent females may be faced with a cultural mandate for which they are ill prepared and which runs counter to their basic psychological dispositions. If women have strong natural needs to secure and maintain interpersonal connections, then requiring them to ignore affiliation and focus instead upon acquiring power might easily produce deep confusion, uncertainty and fear."

Carol Gilligan's theory of female psychology, as set forth in her book *In a Different Voice,* has been cited as reinforcement for these traditional views. She is frequently asked to speak at conferences on eating disorders. Based on her research at Harvard, Gilligan emphasizes women's view of life as essentially different from men's and stresses that it should not be measured against the male model of development. She points out that complex factors make attachment and affiliation with others a major developmental need among women, while men are motivated toward autonomy and individuation.

In our view, Gilligan's research is being misinterpreted. Theorists in eating disorders are ignoring contemporary realities. When we joined the Cornell community twenty years ago, few women were studying to be veterinarians, lawyers, and engineers. Now the picture has changed, and a significant percentage of graduates in these three professional schools are women. It would be unrealistic to suggest these women give up the power and status they have achieved and strive for the type of affiliation that seems to suggest immersion in the roles of wife and mother. Affiliation with men in the traditional sense has become more and more problematic for women. The number of single women aged eighteen to thirty living alone has tripled in the last ten years. One out of five women today *has no potential mate* because there are simply not enough single men to go around, and the situation intensifies as women get older. There are twice as many single women in their forties as there are single men of the same age. Even if affiliation with men is a basic and necessary feminine need, it may remain unfulfilled for some time (perhaps forever!). *Adaptability, patience,* and *self-growth* represent alternative healthy solutions. Affiliation need not be defined only in relationship to men. Women have greater appreciation now for the concept of sisterhood, for the value of friendship among women, and for networking. As Rita Freedman emphasizes in her book *Beauty Bound:* "In friendship, women can support each other (as they are used to supporting men) by encouraging, complimenting, admiring, nurturing, sustaining, celebrating. In effect, sisterhood can provide a 'bulwark against foot binding.' "

We believe it is not the feminist movement but rather the diluting of feminist values that has contributed to the epidemic of eating disorders. Sadly, a majority of white middle-class women of the eighties lack a collective spirit. There is a strong feminist backlash that we observe consistently in our college audiences. Marlene is often told not to identify herself as a feminist for fear no one will attend her lectures. Academics have told her that women's studies programs in colleges have decreased. Gloria Steinem and other feminists express their dismay at the apathy and conservatism of today's young women.

Jane Fonda often is blamed for "aerobic nervosa," the obsessive pursuit of thinness via fitness. Some researchers even maintain that the pursuit of fitness may have become another weapon in the arsenal of rigid weight control, leading to eating disorders. In our view, strenuous exercise is a necessary component of healthful living, and the benefits of exercise for fitness far outweigh potential dangers. While we probably won't convince women to immediately gain the fifteen pounds they may need, we must provide healthy alternatives to the behavior of purging as a means of weight control. Strenuous exercise guides women to new, more self-enhancing ways to experience their bodies. Rather than concentrating on dreaded calories, women now have the opportunity to experience feelings of power, strength, mastery, and enhanced self-concept.

The majority of women with eating disorders lack experience, confidence, and security in their "masculine" endeavors, and this leads them to cling desperately to the feminine ideals of beauty and slimness. It confines them but feels safe, as Rita Freedman points out: "Beauty provides women with a ready-made identity. . . . Without beauty to define us, how can we be women? . . . Women cling to the beauty role because they feel they have much to gain from it: the security of a familiar image; the pleasure of flattery; an achievement arena that does not evoke fear of success; a rationalization for failure; a source of power to attract and influence others; a pleasant diversion and a way to fill time; an excuse to postpone decisions while waiting for Mr. Right. . . . These are the rewards that keep us wed to a mythical beauty ideal. These are the losses we fear when faced with the challenge of change."

With such conflict and confusion over role identity, it is scarcely coincidental that the two uniquely feminine disorders—anorexia and bulimarexia—became widespread in the seventies and continue to engage our attention today.

NOW let's take a closer look at the families of these women, with particular attention to the typical family constellation that can lead to the development of bulimarexic behavior.

"Mom is the villain." Overwhelmingly, this has been the conclusion whenever eating disorders in children are examined. Researchers and clinicians, and even feminist writers, are likely to hold mothers responsible; all deplore the controlling mother, who is seen as "perfectionistic, domineering, and overinvolved" with her children.

The literature continues to emphasize the influence of mothers on daughters. Girls are said to be raised by mothers who reject their own bodies, thereby perpetuating a legacy of anxiety and self-loathing. At a recent conference on eating disorders in New York City, author Susie Orbach asserted that a mother's inconsistency of response to a daughter is a "failure of maternal nurturance." Thus, Orbach continues where Hilde Bruch left off, in attributing child pathology to maternal pathology and in relating eating disorders to bad or inconsistent mothering.

This entrenched view is myopic, destructive, and unjust. In the area of eating disorders, mothers' overinvolvement in the lives of their daughters is rarely viewed as stemming from the same frustrations and feelings of helplessness and powerlessness that their daughters experience. Many experts evidence a total lack of compassion for these mothers, an almost self-righteous, across-the-board condemnation that fails to take into account the complexities involved in these mother-daughter relationships.

Typically, the mothers of our bulimarexics were women who abandoned careers (or never embarked on them) in order to raise children. Initially, they gloried in their motherhood. The commitment to their families and homes was their means of personal fulfillment, and they subscribed to the view that children could not grow to full potential without a mother's constant attention and care. Like the college classmates Betty Friedan wrote about in *The Feminine Mystique,* these mothers made painful transitions into middle age. The vicarious gratification attained by way of a husband's achievement or the accomplishments of children no longer sustained them. Many grew increasingly disillusioned, depressed, and neurotic. Outwardly dominant, but inwardly weak and unhappy, these mothers felt ineffectual in most areas of their lives. Since they were married to men who were generally preoccupied with their careers, or "out to lunch," as one of our women put it, these mothers exercised "authority by default" over their children. At times they were suffocating and overbearing, as if to compensate for their powerlessness elsewhere.

Putting the blame on mothers may afford a certain satisfaction, in that mothers are punished for past transgressions, but it is especially destructive for bulimarexics. The young women then are focusing their energy on the past as they seek the underlying reasons for their compulsive eating habits. They are concentrating on the *whys* rather than on *what they are gaining* from such behavior patterns. Once women come to realize that they have embraced the same legacy of helplessness and hopelessness that their mothers have lived out, they can free themselves to choose a different way of living. They can reject what they perceive as frivolous, demeaning, and irrational and develop skills that are fulfilling and growth enhancing. The problem for many daughters is that in their attempts to move away from their mothers' legacy, they do not move toward other alternatives (except food). Daughters who cling to the belief that they are "tragic victims" who can only control their lives through food deny themselves the joys and pains of growth and the opportunity to develop competence, self-reliance, and independence. In blaming their mothers, they absolve themselves from personal responsibility and remain locked in the past, paralyzed in the present, and fearful of the future. They do not see their mothers as victims too and fail to understand or appreciate the pain and conflict that molded them.

Assuming the role of victim can have other disastrous consequences. Rather than rejecting the passive-aggressive behavior of their mothers, many of the bulimarexics we have treated struggle for a social acceptance that would allow them to reenact their mothers' roles. Again, since they cannot imagine that there are alternatives, their only option appears to be to follow in their mothers' footsteps. The resulting and mutually demoralizing dependency results in further powerlessness for both mother and daughter. In overt and covert ways, the mother transmits her frustration at being a woman; the daughter, in turn, feels hopeless about her own future.

In our initial work with bulimarexic women, we too were caught up in stereotypical assumptions about mother-daughter strife, especially since many of our women were involved with struggles for independence. However, we soon learned that some of the women took issue with the condemnation of "mother as villain" and were upset by Marlene's first article about bulimarexia in *Signs,* which reiterated this theme. On the contrary, these women argued, they loved their mothers. In order to gain more insight into these responses, we began to administer detailed family history questionnaires to our group members and were surprised at what we learned. Taking into consideration the bulimarexic's characteristic inability to express open anger and the fact that she may not be able to express her feelings honestly, there were nonetheless a number of women who said they loved their mothers unconditionally. Of the first 120 Cornell coeds polled, 55 percent characterized their relationships with their mothers as good. The following examples are typical:

"She has always had my interests at heart and tried to teach me independence. She's strong and smart."

"Our relationship has been very close; she has been loving to all her children. I feel very much like her, and we understand each other very well."

Others spoke of relationships, once stormy, that were improving with time.

In addition to the 55 percent who described their relationships with their mothers as good, 40 percent said they felt ambivalent. They both loved and hated their mothers. On the one hand, they could respect their mothers for their ability to juggle multiple roles and could admire their physical beauty or social competence. On the other hand, they had scorn for their mothers' weaknesses, rages, and/or breakdowns. They swung from love to hate and felt guilt during "hate cycles." Some even felt that they had to protect their mothers from depression. The comment of one woman sums it up: "If I start to live, she'll start to die! Guilt! I was a great Mama's girl, very close. She is an all-too-loving woman—she overparents me and is manipulative. I hate and love her. We fight a lot. She demands to know my feelings and then tells me my feelings are wrong. She's depressed a lot."

These women also resent the way their mothers submit to the domination of husbands: "After I became a teenager, I had little respect for my mother because I thought she would never stand up to my father." Another woman expressed herself in a similar way. The words she uses clearly illustrate her ambivalence: "We get along well, and we get along much better now than in the past. I do feel my mother lets my father dominate her too much. She works for him for no salary and waits on him hand and foot. I love her but feel sorry for her when she lets my father push her around."

In our experience, many bulimarexic women are likely to have approach-avoidance conflicts with their mothers. While they may despise their mothers at times and resent the suffocation of their overinvolvement, they nonetheless often seek their mothers' support. They love and admire them for certain qualities; they compete with them, feel sorry for them, and confide in them. In fact, the bulimarexic woman's relationship with her mother is often her only source of support in a closed and alienated nuclear family where the father is distant, either physically or emotionally or both.

For the most part, bulimarexic women do not express overt hostility toward their fathers. However, some of the same women who told us that they loved their mothers said that their fathers were the problem! It is interesting that few investigators have addressed the father's role in childhood disorders, particularly with regard to eating disorders. This obviously has to do with the status accorded the fathers as breadwinners who are preoccupied with their careers and who carry on the important and necessary work of men in the world outside the family. As Phyllis Chesler points out in *Women and Madness:* "Fathers invade children too (their privacy and selves, etc.), but not as frequently. They don't have to. They already own the entire territory and need only make occasional forays to check on their holdings."

The impact of these remote fathers can have far-reaching consequences for the family as a whole. Mothers generally take up the reins with bitterness when fathers relinquish their responsibilities. Although these mothers may appear dominant—at least in the home and over their children—they remain submissive to their husbands in all other realms. For it is the fathers who hold the economic bargaining power. And, as already indicated, the mothers exercise authority by default.

Paternal rejection and secret yearnings for intimacy with their fathers were evident in the history of many of the bulimarexics we treated. According to these daughters, lack of intimacy with their fathers was as much responsible for their feelings of inadequacy and lack of self-esteem as were the strife-ridden relationships with their mothers. A surprising 47 percent of our 120 coeds characterized their relationships with Dad as bad! Anger at him, when they were able to release it, was more vehemently expressed than that aimed at mothers. The following quotes illustrate the pain many women feel because of the unavailability of fathers:

"Daddy was always at work. Occasionally he noticed me. Usually he put me down. I hate him."

"Messed up! My father always traveled and was away more than he was home. He left us for two years to live in Europe."

"He is very reserved and never emotional. I can only communicate with him on a superficial basis. I have harbored deep resentment for my father and the pain he has caused my family."

Several women described their fathers as tyrannical and had always been frightened of their anger. One called her father "irresponsible, domineering, and crazy. I stay away from him." Another said her father "rules the household with an iron hand. He's an autocrat, a little Hitler; we never talk." Others were fearful of the variability of their fathers' moods.

Occasionally the daughters have some insight into how the behavior of father and mother feed into a family system that is damaging to all members. The daughter of a successful lawyer has this to say: "He will do anything for a client. As a father he leaves me empty. My father never hugs and kisses me. He hides his emotions and told me one had to hide one's emotions. My mother dropped out of college during her third year. A society belle, she married my father. There is no communication. We have a destructive relationship, and I am ever dependent on them. They are my social life."

The following statement is even more perceptive: "My father is very insecure. He depends on his children to fulfill certain needs in his life and takes very personally the things that we do that may or may not fulfill needs in his life. He's very critical of me. My mother plays an interesting subordinate role but actually runs the family and is the dominant one. She allows my father to think that *he* does, however, because he needs to feel that."

In contrast to the closeness that had evolved over the years with mothers, many women felt that their relationships with their fathers were deteriorating. The high school or college years were pinpointed as the beginning of this change for the worse: "We had a loving and trusting relationship until the last few years," one woman said. "I can see through his idealistic crap now. He doesn't practice what he preaches." While this comment might reflect the young woman's general maturation, most women related their conflicts with fathers to their first steps toward separation from the family. At this time, some fathers seemed to want them to stay little girls or, at least, to accept the traditional feminine role. Here are some indicative comments:

"For the most part, he favored me and loved me a lot . . . but he turned away from me during adolescence. He emphasized my looks, yet praised others for their mind and talent."

"We got along together in high school, much better than my mother and I, but since I've gone to college, my father and I don't get along so well. He still treats me like a little girl, but he'd like to see me get married."

"During high school he tried to make me into a female domestic . . . after years of encouraging independence and exploring interests!"

It might not be stretching it too much to say that these fathers encouraged and supported their daughters while they lived under the fathers' roofs, but once the young women made efforts toward independence, fathers encouraged them to become like their mothers.

Whatever criticism they had, many of the bulimarexic women we questioned idolized their fathers. Fathers were viewed as successful and powerful, and their attention and approval, intermittent as it might be, was valued more than the love they received from their mothers. When they felt their fathers withdrawing, they often tried harder to please them, usually without success. And so the ground was laid for the lifelong quest for male approval (often associated with physical perfection). This wistful statement from one of our women is indicative of the feelings of many: "My father is somewhat of a maverick—very successful and very much the outdoor sportsman and athlete. I tried so hard to emulate him and be his favorite."

Often the time when fathers withdrew from their daughters coincided with a move toward their growing sons. Another familial theme running through the histories of women with eating disorders is the intense competition they experience with siblings. Fifty-eight percent of the coeds sampled in our initial survey had older brothers, and more often than not the brother was the favored child. Our women soon found that no matter how perfect or successful they were, the accomplishments of brothers were regarded more highly. They were learning "how to feel small," with the accompanying lesson that "good girls don't win ball games." What's more, the parental expectations for female and male children were quite different.

"Our parents had distinct aspirations for both me and my brother," one woman said. "He was encouraged to accomplish great feats in the world. I was just supposed to be happy, marry well, and love my children. There was the expectation he would pursue a career. It never occurred to them (or me) that I might someday have to support myself."

Some families discriminated in a more overt manner. In the following comment, when competition developed between a brother and sister, the girl was effectively muzzled, beginning at an early age:

I have a brother who is fifteen months younger than I am who at a very early age started to have psychological problems. A child psychiatrist told my parents that it was due to the fact that he was competing with me and I was always achieving. If something would break, I would fix it, for example. So, when I was about five or six, the psychiatrist told my parents that the competition was too much. I was deflating his male ego and they should try to separate us a little bit so that we weren't in competition so much. And the way my parents dealt with that was to tell me to try to stop doing better than him all the time. They asked me, don't fix it if it breaks, let him do it. They sort of asked me not to succeed and to succeed at the same time. From that time on, I've had the confusion of wanting to do well, but then being afraid that it wasn't OK to do well.

Thus we can see how maternal overprotection, paternal censure and deprivation, as well as rivalry with siblings (generally male) can propel a young woman toward the kind of stress that can result in eating disorders. We must, however, avoid the pitfall of relying on categories that are too neat, or we run the risk of creating new stereotypes. When we extended our initial treatment of bulimarexic college students to women of all ages and walks of life, we encountered many women who claimed that they loved and respected both parents. Their fathers, they said, were supportive and loving, and many of the mothers had achieved success in careers. Yet, although the family atmosphere had been more harmonious, these daughters typically had been overprotected. Most of them had not acquired the skills to cope with the world beyond the safe walls of the home. Raised to believe they were the "best," they learned to expect lavish praise and encouragement, but they had little experience with failure and rejection. And when they left home for college, their families were no longer there to envelop them with the protection they had grown to require.

Let us now turn to adolescence and the pressures that impinge on young women *outside* the family.

4.

Adolescence: Setting the Stage for Eating Disorders

SEVENTEEN magazine, in January 1982, featured an article entitled "Do You Stuff Yourself One Moment and Starve Yourself the Next?" The article introduced the magazine's readership—thousands of adolescent girls—to the binge/purge eating disorder. In a section of the article called "Where to Go for Help," our names were mentioned. Once again we received a dismaying number of letters. We no longer underestimated the epidemic nature of the syndrome and so were not particularly surprised at the amount of mail. However, to receive letters from girls who had not reached puberty—some of them only ten years old!—gave us a new and shocking perspective.

One preteen told us with fear and even a bit of pride that her mother had not caught on yet to the fact that she made herself throw up four or five times a day "after eating everything in sight." Another girl, in her midteens, confessed that she had "bulimia, but not real bad." She had been vomiting once or twice a day for a year or so. A third complained, "No one will take me seriously. I know I am fat. Everyone says I'm just saying that to get attention, and they tell me I'm crazy." This girl added wistfully, "I guess they think I will outgrow it. I have tried to stop but can't."

For Marlene, the mother of teenage twin daughters, the letters were especially painful. She remembered all too clearly an incident that had taken place when Debbie and Becky were twelve. It was an incident that could have propelled the girls toward eating problems similar to the ones we are now writing about.

Marlene had always encouraged the twins to participate in sports, an experience she had missed when she was a young girl in the fifties. (At that time, boys typically engaged in strenuous physical activity, while girls dabbled at dance exercises and played volleyball.) At the age of twelve the twins had solid, trim bodies and were proficient in several sports. Gymnastics was the favorite, and they particularly liked their mother to watch them perform. Marlene literally wrote portions of her dissertation at the gymnastics center as the twins learned one routine after another.

At the end of the class, Marlene generally took the girls to the local Tastee Freeze for ice cream. One evening Debbie was very quiet, unlike her usual animated self, and said she did not want ice cream. No explanation. Marlene waited until they were home to ask what was wrong. Debbie dissolved in tears and said that she hated her body and wished she were dead: "I don't want breasts and I don't want hips. I hate my fat!" she sobbed.

Marlene was thunderstruck. As a feminist she had tried to help both girls develop a positive attitude toward their bodies and their emerging womanhood. Debbie was not fat, by any stretch of the imagination. Now, after treating numerous women suffering from bulimarexia, Marlene was seeing an anorexic-like response in her own healthy daughter.

After gentle prodding, Debbie revealed that her gymnastics coach had triggered her sudden loathing for her body. The coach had pointed to Debbie's stomach, slightly rounded as is normal for twelve-year-olds, and remarked, "You should lose a few pounds." That was all that was said.

Setting aside her role as therapist Marlene reacted emotionally as a mother. In detail she pointed out what she considered to be flaws and imperfections in her own body, and she told the twins that while she might not consider her body type perfect, she would have to be satisfied with certain aspects of it for the rest of her life, no matter what self-restraint, no matter what amount of dieting. She asked the girls to love their bodies and accept the flaws and even invited them to consider her stretch marks, "created by the most beautiful experience I ever had, giving birth to twins."

It was a heady scene, with much crying and hugging, but afterward the girls appeared fortified and stronger. Four years later, Becky faced a similar experience, but handled it differently. She was trying to earn a much-coveted spot on the gymnastic team and to her delight was chosen. Becky was then 5'3" and weighed 110 pounds. Her new coach immediately indicated that she would have to lose from ten to fifteen pounds. Without hesitation, Becky told the coach that losing that much weight would weaken her body and interfere with her performance. She quietly indicated her refusal and quit the team.

Such experiences, unless properly handled, indicate how an irrational fear of being fat can develop. Indeed, the preference for thinness can begin to take hold at a much earlier age, reflecting the preferences of our culture.

In 1978 researchers at the University of Cincinnati College of Medicine examined the attitudes and preferences of preschool-age children in an effort to find the age at which antifat concepts emerge. Overwhelmingly, most (91 percent) preferred a thin rag doll over a fat one. The handful of overweight children in the study also chose the thin doll, although they could not say why. As early as three to five years old, then, there is a certain stigma attached to being overweight, and selective pressures on female children may have already been implanted. Other long-standing childhood studies support the findings that children develop a distinct aversion to chubby bodies and prefer athletic lean ones. In 1967 Dr. J. R. Staffieri of the University of Indiana presented six- to ten-year-old male boys with silhouettes of obese, normal, and thin bodies. Uniformly, the subjects reacted unfavorably to the fatter ones. Furthermore, they attributed disparaging characteristics to the "fatty," labeling it as dirty, lazy, lying, sloppy, mean, ugly, and stupid. In 1972 Staffieri showed the same silhouettes to female children. They too reacted unfavorably to the fatty but added even more negative characteristics to their descriptions of it.

So it seems that both boys and girls disparage fat in childhood; however, beginning with adolescence, females overwhelmingly become more influenced than males. In 1971 Dr. E. Clifford at the

Duke University Medical School found that 194 adolescent females aged eleven to nineteen were more dissatisfied with and critical of their bodies than 146 males of the same age range. A later study at the University of Iowa revealed that girls were beginning to undergo a distortion of body image, believing that they looked quite a bit heavier than they were. Eighty-six girls (ages ten to eighteen) from the Iowa City schools consistently overestimated the girth of their bodies. These studies indicated that young females wanted to be smaller but believed themselves incapable of attaining this ideal. Many experts in eating disorders believe these early childhood attitudes persist and may contribute to self-loathing and poor self-esteem in those who gain weight at later ages and could create extreme self-consciousness in anyone who fears becoming overweight.

The cultural message to be slim is transmitted to the child through many sources—the family, the child's peer group, teachers, books, magazines, and television. Children try to behave in a way that is consistent with the beliefs and behaviors of people in the groups to which they belong. When all groups agree, certain values are introduced without question. In our culture, the message is clear: Slimness is best.

At the same time, there is much to encourage excessive eating and weight gain. An abundance of fast food products exists, and we are bombarded with manipulative advertising from the food industry. Junk foods and fast foods are described as luscious and mouth-watering, with consumers challenged to binge: "Bet you can't eat just one!" Tempting snack foods help us to chew away our leisure hours. The presence of food is tied to recreational events and socializing, with cookouts, clambakes, and picnics part of the American way of life. We are led to snack during movies or while watching television. Children and teenagers are especially susceptible to this kind of advertising.

If both boys and girls disapprove of fat in childhood and yet experience simultaneous conflicting messages to be slim and to eat excessively, what happens in adolescence to escalate this hatred of fat and self in girls? The answer seems to lie in the socialization rituals to which both sexes, but particularly women, are exposed. What are these socialization rituals and how are they conveyed? What are the subtle as well as overt pressures that encourage smallness of mind and body in adolescent girls?

Adolescence has always been an emotionally difficult passage, with youngsters typically feeling isolated, different, and out-of-step. Dr. Peter Blos, author of several books on adolescent passage, views this stage of life as a "struggle to regain a psychic equilibrium which has been jolted by the crisis of puberty." Blos believes the basic task of the adolescent is to arrive at a subjective feeling that "this is my way of life." A failure to achieve this sense can lead to adaptive failures and even severe psychopathology. Erik Erikson stresses these same major points in his developmental theory.

In our culture, the problem is that "identity" involves different goals and expectations for boys and girls as they move away from their primary identity of child and toward adolescence. Caryl Rivers, Rosalind Barnett, and Grace Baruch emphasize this point in their book *Beyond Sugar and Spice: How Women Grow, Learn and Thrive.* "Boys aim high—they look at the stars. Girls seem to peer up to the lowest branch in a nearby tree." (And, we might add, cling to it for dear life.) For boys, signposts along the road to masculine identity have always been clear and well-defined. "To be a man" implies strength of character, courage, and the willingness to take risks and become independent. Until recent years, "to be a woman" meant serving and caring for other people. Men were taught to be outwardly directed and "to make a go of it" before settling down and taking on new responsibilities and obligations. Men have been conditioned to move away from their original families and to find primary fulfillment through work. Women, on the other hand, have been directed away from their families of birth to form new families in which caring for husbands and children has been expected to provide the ultimate fulfillment. In *Beyond Sugar and Spice,* the authors sum up adolescent passage as the time when boys become men by doing and girls become women by finding a man.

Self-concept evolves through social interaction and is largely a product of socialization. There is now evidence that parents, especially fathers, regard their male and female infants in different ways based solely on the infant's gender. Although infant girls may weigh more at birth and actually be hardier than comparable boy infants, they are still viewed as weaker and more fragile.

When children enter nursery school, teachers often react differently to boys and girls. One study of nursery-school children reported that girls were encouraged to cling and ask many questions, while boys were taught to do and to be active. Other researchers report a sharp rise in "people orientedness" among girls at about the age of ten. Throughout adolescence, girls are more dependent than boys on the favorable opinions of others. Self-consciousness (as opposed to a sense of self) increases in girls and decreases in boys as they begin to mature.

Success experiences in adolescence are, of course, crucial in developing a sense of confidence and self-esteem. However, researchers have found that girls begin to value *interpersonal success* more than boys at this time. Girls depend so much for their identities on relationships with others, especially boys, that rejection can be devastating. Boys certainly experience rejection in relationships, but they are in the process of forming identities that can sustain them. The young male is admonished to "act like a man" when disappointed and to "pick himself up" and carry on. By the time boys reach adolescence, they have had much more experience dealing with criticism, defeat, and rejection. Witness any typical adolescent dance! The boys are lined up on one side of the dance floor, the girls on the other. The twelve-year-old boy ventures across the floor as his male friends watch carefully. When he reaches the chosen girl, he asks her to dance. She refuses. Amid the hoots and jeers of his peers, the young boy must traverse the endless distance back to his friends. He may feel little and small, but he does not *act* it. His socialization has already taught him that men do not allow themselves to be brought down by such experiences.

Girls, on the other hand, are reinforced for dependent and

approval-seeking behavior. With little experience in developing confidence and autonomy, they carry a greater fear of rejection than do boys. This fear, when combined with an obsessive preoccupation with boys, can become a prominent and primary psychological characteristic of adolescent girls, leading to irrational and crippling fantasies about their own fragility, helplessness, and powerlessness. Confidence in being able to cope with their environment is thus eroded by such paralyzing fears and expectations related to the horrors of rejection.

In almost all aspects of a young woman's life, then, the answer to "What is my identity?" is fraught with negative associations. The period of adolescence for women has been described as a "dropping back" time, a turning away from individual achievement and competition toward what Jean Lipman Blumen, of the National Institute of Education, describes as "the Vicarious Achievement Ethic." Perhaps this settling for less was revealed in an important 1978 study conducted by John C. Condry and Sharon L. Dyer of Cornell. Sixty-one children in the fifth, seventh, and ninth grades were given what were described as intelligence tests. Boys were assigned girl partners and were seated across from them. Each boy and girl was then taken aside and told that he or she had done better than his or her partner: "You won—you were five points better!" The youngsters were then given a second chance at the test. The researchers had set up this situation to test what they predicated would be a "sudden onset" of fear of success among girls in *mixed sex* competition at the time of puberty—the time when beliefs about "sex appropriate" behaviors are apparently formed. The results were illuminating. Both male and female fifth grade students increased their scores on the test the second time around. However, between the fifth and seventh grade, a radically different pattern emerged. Seventh grade boys increased their scores, while 80 percent of the girls dropped their scores after being told that they had bested a male partner. To a lesser degree, the same was true for the ninth grade girls. When they were asked about their test responses, most seventh grade girls—those at the onset of puberty—revealed a reluctance to compete with boys, especially to beat them at games. One ray of hope lay with the second group of ninth grade girls, who did not drop their scores. They felt they should always try their best no matter what the circumstances!

Mary Pipher (1994) believes that something dramatic is happening to adolescent girls in the 1990s and that they are having many more problems now than ten or twenty years ago! Preadolescent girls between seven and eleven are fairly well-adjusted and happy. Then something dramatic happens to them in early adolescence, causing their IQ scores to drop. They become less curious and more deferential and self-critical—especially about their bodies. They also become depressed. Pipher views the diluting of feminist values and the lip service paid to equality as a compelling factor. Add this to the growing *social problems* of more divorced families, chemical addictions, casual sex, and the explosion of sexually transmitted diseases, as well as violence against women and soft- and hard-core pornography, and we are witnessing unprecedented stress on youngsters with a suicide rate among children aged ten to fourteen rising over 75 percent between 1979 and 1988. It is not "changing roles for women" that creates stress, misery, eating disorders, and other adolescent struggles. Girls are also subjected to increasing physical and sexual assaults, are more vulnerable, less secure, and more likely to have experienced upheaval and trauma in their lives, and are less free to strike out on their own in a landscape resembling a battlefield where date rape, herpes, AIDS, and drive-by shootings have become commonplace. Old stressors combine with new ones, creating suffering for all adolescent girls, not just those with eating disorders. It is not just the often quoted cliché of "the fear of growing up" that is the problem but the reality of growing up in a society that is clearly hostile, dangerous, and damaging to women. The girls and women I work with are very clear about their goals and excited about their choices and opportunities. The majority do not appear to be suffering from role confusion. It is not their *future dreams* that are causing conflict. It is their present state of starvation that is the major problem.

Many existing studies of depression in children support Pipher's clinical observations. Preadolescent children either evidence no gender differences in rates of depression or boys are somewhat more likely to be depressed than girls. Then sometime around the ages of thirteen to fourteen girls consistently begin to show higher rates of depression than boys, as much as two to one. The greater female rate of depression then continues throughout the lifespan for every adult age group except the elderly (Nolen-Hoeksema 1990).

Susan Nolen-Hoeksema (1995) identifies a feminine style of *coping* and proposes that throughout adolescence and adulthood women tend to have a more ruminative and passive style of responding to their own distress than men. This style of mood management exacerbates and prolongs periods of distress that arise for women and interfere with a woman's ability to overcome the negative events they face.

Sethi and Nolen-Hoeksemsa in their study "Gender Differences in Internal and External Focusing Among Adolescents" (1997) found striking gender differences in *nondepressed* youngsters. Girls devoted more thoughts to thinking about themselves and the people they know (internally and relationally focused). Boys, in contrast, displayed a tendency toward external focusing, thinking about everything else such as sports, music, and food even when asked to talk about themselves. They preferred to engage in positive thoughts regardless of the condition they were in. Girls, on the other hand, ruminate whether they are satisfied or frustrated. What is particularly relevant is the finding that depressed and nondepressed females share a similar style of coping that seems to be present by early adolescence.

Some of the biological and social challenges of adolescence that seem to enhance the development of eating disorders may be body dissatisfaction and pressure to conform to restrictive social roles deemed appropriate for females (Rierdan et al. 1988). Many researchers have argued that both boys and girls who are dissatisfied with their bodies are more likely to become depressed (Brooks-Gunn 1988, Rierdan et al. 1988). Beginning in puberty, however, girls become more dissatisfied and thus more prone to depression.

McCarthy (1990) suggests the more negative body image of girls leads many towards chronic dieting that *in itself* contributes to helplessness and depression.

In a series of studies of sixth, eighth, and tenth grade students, researchers found evidence that girls who accept a narrowing of activities and interests prescribed by the feminine gender role were at risk for higher levels of depressive symptoms (Girgus et al. 1989; Girgus, Nolen-Hoeksema, Paul, and Spears 1991). Girls in sixth through tenth grades who spent more time in feminine-type activities—shopping, beauty rituals, and the like—exhibited higher depressive symptomology. On the other hand, those girls who resisted were rejected by peers. Showing one's competence and otherwise violating feminine stereotypes also led to depression (Block, Gjerde, and Block 1991). Thus, these girls encounter consistent double-bind, or "catch-22," situations in which no matter what they do they cannot win.

Researchers found that the more intelligent girls were, the more depressed they were. Girls increasingly want to conceal their intelligence as they go through adolescence (Rosen and Aneshensel 1976). This may explain the drop in IQ scores that Pipher has pointed out. More recent data find girls are still more concerned than boys about *others'* judgments of their appearance and behaviors (Nolen-Hoeksema and Larson 1992). Thus, it makes more sense to blame *femininity*, not feminism for the these higher ratios of depression and eating disorders in girls.

One other important aspect of adolescence that must be mastered is the ability to form new and more mature relationships with one's own age group. Here again current research suggests that adolescent friendships among males reinforce movement toward activity and achievement while girls, fearful of being on their own, tend to cling to each other. While boys use friends as allies in efforts to break away from authority, girls often form intense conformist alliances, which researcher Janet Lever has referred to as "mini marriages." Much of their conversation centers around how to snare this boy or that one—in short, there is an excessive, often obsessional, amount of thinking about boys.

Identity is often described by contemporary social scientists as *the things one does,* and the need is emphasized for several identities—some vocational and some recreational. The amount of success experienced in each of these identities determines self-concept. When successes outnumber failures, there is a reasonable chance that a positive identity will be formed. If a young girl's identity is so closely tied to successes in interpersonal relationships (which are typically transient and short-lived at this age), it is not difficult to see how the adolescent girl can develop a negative or "nothing" identity. Brothers and boyfriends are, of course, extremely interested in girls, but their energies are directed into other pursuits as well. They are forming positive attitude toward their growing bodies by developing them and feeling the strength and power of their maleness. This positive acceptance of one's body is also consistently cited as another crucial developmental task to be mastered in adolescence. While boys may find the changes in their bodies as disturbing and disorienting as girls do the changes in their own, they rarely view the changes as crippling or subtracting from their self-concept—quite the contrary, as Rivers and her colleagues point out, they are "badges of manhood."

A special rite of passage for women involves the onset of menstruation. There is ample evidence that adolescent girls, even today, have negative feelings about their bodies as they begin their menstrual cycle. A major study conducted in 1978 by Anne E. Clarke and Diane Ruble of Princeton found overwhelming evidence that both female and male adolescents entertain very negative beliefs about menstruation. Over 50 percent of the girls worried that someone would know they were having their periods. Further, both sexes equated menstruation with emotionality and with disruption of activities as well as performance in school. Judith Bardwick, a psychologist at the University of Michigan, begins an essay about women's psychological conflict and the reproductive system by stating: "To a very large extent women are their bodies." It would not be too extreme to add that women become prisoners of their bodies as well. The following is a beautiful but unfortunately rare attempt on the part of one family to reverse these crippling socialization rituals. In her book *Menstruation and Menopause,* Paula Weideger cites a letter she received from parents: "We have two daughters, twelve and seven. The twelve-year-old just had her first menstruation. We drank wine and toasted her. Her father gave her a bunch of wildflowers. She seemed pleased and open."

In our view, the general inability of adolescent girls to take pride in their bodies is one important reason why they have great difficulty establishing identities as women. Few realize that females are more durable physically than males. Consider that the female must be strong enough to nourish and carry the fetus through the prenatal period in order to insure the survival of the species. During the course of evolution, it is hypothesized that stronger females survived, while males, whose role in procreation does not require that kind of strength and endurance, were not selected for those qualities. The *myth of feminine fragility* must be banished, and young women must learn to identify positively with their bodies. This includes accepting and embracing changes that take place in the body. The bloating and weight gain that often accompany menstruation need not be viewed as unbearable. The pregnant female body, often associated with "unattractive changes" and the belief that "I will never have a perfect body again," should engender feelings of joy, power, and uniqueness, not self-loathing.

Emerging sexuality can also create enormous conflict in young women and increase the fear and distrust they have about their bodies. While they may be physically capable of the sexual act, few are ready for it emotionally. Our current mores present special problems. No longer is there the proscription to "save one's virginity." The so-called sexual revolution of the sixties did away with this important psychological protection. (To be fair, it was a proscription accepted by young men as well, at least as far as the "girls they were going to marry" were concerned.) Today the pressure to have early sexual experiences is intense and unrelenting. Understandably, many young women begin to think of themselves as victims. This feeling coincides with the time when they are beginning to receive special attention because of external attractiveness. All around, there are pressures that perpetuate the image of woman as ornamental, with her body the main commodity of worth. And behind this is the ultimate fantasy of attracting and capturing a man. Thus, "going along with him" and the "fear of losing him" can create overwhelming anxieties. The young girl is already learning to adapt to the desires and needs of others and, in effect, makes her own transformation into a sexual object.

Advertisements further convince us that this is how women are or want to be. According to sociologists Gloria I. Joseph and Jill Lewis, advertising creates and shapes our values and fears so that we come to believe that imposed values/fears/attitudes/goals are our own, as if we had chosen them. In 1982 Joseph and Lewis conducted a survey of leading women's magazines to determine how female sex roles are presented and portrayed and to explore recurrent themes. They found that beauty ads comprised 68 percent of all advertising in *Cosmopolitan* magazine, and most women were portrayed as sexy, subordinate, and seductive, as competitors with other women, and as dependent on men. These researchers concluded:

The purpose of such institutionalized sexism operates in advertising for the purpose of maintaining the image of women as dependent sex objects who are inferior and subordinate to men. Consumerism is therefore promoted by keeping women in a constant state of self-doubt and self-denigration. They are constantly admonished to aspire to impossible standards of beauty and sexuality by spending. The selling of the image of woman as a sex object is big business and results in women competing against one another to achieve this illusionary image.

In 1977 sociologist Erving Goffman of the University of Pennsylvania observed that advertisements tended to show men as physically elevated above women, therefore reinforcing the image of women as deferential and dependent. In order to pursue these findings further, in 1978 Dane Archer and his associates at the University of California at Santa Cruz examined a total of 1,750 published photographs from *Time, Newsweek, Ms.,* and a number of newspapers. They found a pronounced tendency in all publications to emphasize the faces of men and the bodies of women. Their conclusion was that this was a clear reflection of the tendency to slight the intellectual qualities of women.

Since childhood, female children have been exposed through schoolbooks to portrayals of women in ways that are stereotyped and limited. In 1972 Lenore Weitzman and her colleagues at Yale conducted a study of award-winning preschool picture books and concluded:

Little boys receive attention and praise for their achievements and cleverness. For girls, achievement is marriage and becoming a mother. Most of the women in picture books have status by virtue of their relationships to specific men—they are wives of the kings, judges, adventurers and explorers, but they, themselves, are not the rulers, judges, adventurers and explorers. Through picture books, girls are taught to have low aspirations because there are so few opportunities portrayed as available to them. . . . Women . . . can achieve only by being attractive, congenial and serving others.

Educator D. B. Graebner studied five hundred stories presented in elementary school readers over a ten-year period and reported similar findings in an article published in 1972. Men and boys outnumbered females in the newer editions, and role stereotypes were, if anything, *stronger* in spite of the new feminist awareness of the sixties and seventies. Boys continued to be portrayed as clever, brave, creative, and resourceful, while girls were docile, kind, dependent, and self-abrogating.

Television has become a major influence in the lives of children and also a major means of transmitting the values of society. Many social scientists are quick to point out that the recent wave of feminism has had an impact on television programming, and we can observe it, too. Women are now portrayed as doctors, lawyers, even truck drivers and display strength of character and courage. However, many commercials continue to portray women as insipid, mindless creatures, which may subtract from the influence of the new models of womanhood. Certainly, the commercials for sportswear carry a promise of all good things if the wearer is slim and a threat of failure if she is not.

Additionally, program material on television continues to reinforce a terror of being fat. Well-known actresses who over the years have appeared in movies and on television are significantly slimmer today. Some even appear too thin and unhealthy. One time, on several segments of *The Tonight Show,* almost without exception when women were conversing with each other, the focus was on dieting and the need to lose weight or on weight-related matters. One newly arrived South American singer remarked that she had left the poverty of her country for the United States "in order to eat." Now, after considerable struggle to get here, she had discovered that "she cannot eat!"

Drs. Susan and Orland Wooley, experts on obesity at the University of Cincinnati Medical School, have commented about a television commercial that depicts a fat woman bludgeoning her meek husband with her purse because he did not buy a motorcycle. In another sequence, a macho man who did buy one rides by with a slim young woman clinging to his back. They use this example to illuminate how fat people are ridiculed and ostracized by the media. Occasionally, a more compassionate portrait of an overweight person does find its way to the TV screen. However, the compassion conveyed is often dissipated by the simplistic behavior of the characters, who are almost always stereotypes. Such was the case with "Dinky Hocker," an ABC afterschool television special about an obese adolescent girl, which was shown a number of years ago. Dinky had friends who genuinely cared about her, including boys. She also managed to have fun in social situations. Predictably, however, she dealt with her discomfort about her obesity by overachieving academically and filling her life with hobbies and animals.

Although the film captured Dinky's life in a sensitive and realistic way—i.e., you genuinely felt Dinky's pain and liked her—it was superficial and myopic. From the onset, there was no doubt that it was all Mom's fault. Dinky's mother was portrayed as vicious, obsessed with her life as a committee woman, preoccupied, domineering, overbearing, hysterical, and unfeeling. She referred to Dinky's excess weight as "baby fat" and pushed food on her when she was attempting to diet; she interfered with and effectively sabotaged Dinky's first relationship with a caring boyfriend; she persisted in calling the girl Dinky instead of using her real name, Susan; and she ignored Dinky's weak and pathetic requests for more time and attention. Dinky almost always turned to food after some rejection or confrontation with her mother.

Dinky's father was weak, kindly, passive, and ineffectual. He basked in the glow of his wife's community efforts and spent most of his time as a referee between mother and daughter. While it is clear that he was as distant and remote from Dinky as her mother, the film gave little indication that there was anything lacking in the quality of this father-daughter relationship. His problems with Dinky were never explored or challenged. Rather, the film appeared to accept his passivity unconditionally.

After a major crisis in the family, Mom came to her senses and realized that Dinky's pain was all her fault and that she had better stay home with Dinky where she belonged. The film ended with mother and daughter embracing, as Dad stood by, smiling in his casual, benevolent way.

Along with such antiobesity propaganda, there are extraordinary cultural persuasions to diet. We have come to believe that all life's problems can be solved by dropping pounds. Promises of success, transformation, an end to existential pain, and living happily ever after prevail. Myriad women (and some men) make a fetish of being thin and follow one reducing diet after another without knowing or caring that they can do so only at the price of severe anxiety and persistent health problems. Until very recently, being underweight was not considered as dangerous nutritionally as being overweight. Dr. Hilde Bruch believes that chronic malnutrition resulting from an abnormal preoccupation with weight is common but not readily recognized as abnormal because it appears under the guise of desirable slimness. Medical experts are only now beginning to call attention to the health hazards of indiscriminate or fad dieting.

In an editorial for the *International Journal of Eating Disorders* (Spring 1982), entitled "The Beverly Hills Eating Disorder: The Mass Marketing of Anorexia Nervosa," the Wooleys provide a scathing indictment of this best-selling popular diet. Pointing to the serious medical problems that can occur if this diet is followed, they say: "That training in anorexic psychopathology is selling so well holds a message. It is a vote of no confidence in the whole effort by helping professions . . . and it reveals a degree of desperation heretofore unknown. The figures mean that women are so afraid of fat they are no longer willing to wait for a safe scientific method of weight control. . . . The prevailing belief is that no price is too high for thinness, including health."

Jane Brody, health columnist for the *New York Times,* has also spoken out about the dangers of the Beverly Hills Diet and other fad diets. Unfortunately, such condemnation does not appear to budge these books off the best-seller lists, and they proliferate.

With the insidious linkage between attractiveness, success and dieting, it should not be surprising that even young women without severe interpersonal problems become preoccupied with weight in adolescence and engage in competitive and contagious dieting regimes with other young women. For adolescence is the time that the pressure to become popular with boys and to appear feminine is greatest. The implicit cultural belief is that there *must be something wrong* with a girl who gains weight, even though it is not at all unusual for both boys and girls to have some weight gain during adolescence. If youngsters are active and do not develop severe anxiety over weight gain—which fosters the urge to binge—most of them would lose weight in a gradual and safe manner in a relatively short period of time. The exhortation to lose weight comes at a time when food becomes an important aspect of social life (think of pizza parties and clambakes, for instance), creating additional tensions beyond the usual anxiety about heterosexual relationships. All of this can keep a adolescent from enjoying new social experiences in a relaxed and easygoing fashion.

When the concerned parents of an adolescent girl consult physicians or books about overweight and dieting, they may find a reiteration of many of the opinions and beliefs that drove their child to strenuous dieting in the first place. Lest the story of Marlene and her twin daughters seem like an isolated instance, consider the following article, which appeared in the *New York Times.* Here a school system and consulting physicians (save one) join hands to reinforce the pursuit of slimness as the ideal.

FAT GIRLS LOSING OUT ON SCHOOL DRILL TEAM

Great Falls, Mont., Dec. 19 (AP)—A curriculum committee has voted to keep fat girls off a high school drill team, unless they can show they are losing a pound a week.

The ruling, which supported school policy, was made last week, despite an appeal from a parent of a Great Falls High School student who said some girls were drinking mineral oil and taking other drastic measures to lose weight.

One girl, in tears, told the school board committee, "If you don't have a weight problem, you just don't understand." But she admitted that she had not followed the 1,500-calorie diet recommended by Eileen Solberg, adviser to the drill team, the Bisonettes.

Three physicians sent the committee a letter supporting the rule, but a fourth, Dr. Daniel Molloy, said the weight restrictions could be dangerous. He said the pressure placed on the young girls by peers and teachers could result in health problems as they tried to lose weight.

As we can see, overweight is still viewed as "the problem," without regard for the frame of mind or underlying issues that led to the overweight—*if there were any to begin with!*

The women we have worked with describe a variety of different pressures that led to their first decision to diet. A majority were overprotected and unprepared for the new demands posed by socializing with the opposite sex. Their families were self-contained units and the girls, as adolescents, felt isolated and socially insecure. Significantly, few were actually overweight at the time. One woman describes how she felt prior to her first diet: "I was a junior in high school, very desperate—longing for a boyfriend. I had a shallow social life—lived in a fantasy world—had faraway crushes that never materialized, but even so, always felt that I wouldn't be able to handle them if I did. Somehow I believed a loss of eight pounds would magically transform me into the princess."

The wish for magical personality transformation is often associated with expectations of weight loss. Shyness, feelings of inadequacy, confusion about men, and even ignorance will disappear as each pound is shed. The adolescent girl hopes that a new personality will be handed to her without any effort on her part. Sleeping Beauty will be awakened by a kiss!

Many women also say that a rejection (generally by a boy) in adolescence was the traumatic event that precipitated their first diet. More often than not, however, the adolescent girl *fantasizes* that she has been rejected because she is too fat. Most actually never heard this from the boys who had rejected them. For example, the two women whose words follow are certain that their fat resulted in rejection even though they had no real proof that this was the causal factor:

"My first real boyfriend dropped me without any explanation. All I felt then was rage at myself for being so fat and ugly, and I vowed never to be that way again."

And the other says, "I had a boyfriend who dropped me inexplicably, and I tied it to being fat."

Pressures can also emanate from family members. Mothers who are themselves obsessed with dieting may express horror when their daughters gain a few pounds: "My mother made me very conscious of my chubbiness after my last summer at overnight camp (age thirteen). I gained nine pounds and was made to feel ashamed and guilty."

Fathers too can set the wheels in motion. Although their total time spent with daughters may be less than in the mother-daughter relationship, their influence is powerful. Many times their standards of attractiveness for daughters are high, and a chance comment such as "you've put on a little weight" can create a humiliating sense of inadequacy in girls. As one young woman, who desperately wanted to please her father, put it: "Ever since I can remember, I wanted to be thin. Thin was in and fat people just weren't as attractive. I thought my thin cousin was somehow better because she was so slender, and I can remember standing behind her in grade school wishing my legs (which were normal) were as thin as hers. I was absolutely traumatized at age fourteen when my father told me I had a fat ass. Somehow I think I just always wanted to be Daddy's daughter and couldn't bear the thought of losing loving nicknames such as 'little face" or 'little bit.' "

The overwhelming desire to please others coupled with extreme self-criticism is the essence of the problem. Debbie and Becky were especially vulnerable to this type of criticism because they were athletes. A similar vulnerability is evident in young dancers. Dr. L. M. Vincent, author of *Competing with the Sylph: Dancers and the Pursuit of the Ideal Body Form,* is a physician (also a dancer) who has observed many impressionable young dancers forced by the weight obsessive dance subculture into destructive eating patterns. In his book, he describes his anger, frustration, and surprise at seeing a young slim dancer he delights in—"about the healthiest little girl I know"—reduced to tears and instilled with an intense desire to diet by the casual criticism of a dance coach: "Watch your weight."

Once dieting is initiated, the process and the end result become as important as the factors that led to the diet in the first place. Dieting provides a sense of meaning and purpose—a distraction from pain, loneliness, and insecurity. Many girls derive feelings of power from this form of self-denial. Others derive secondary gains for their vigilance. Friends are admiring and in awe of the self-denial required to lose weight. "Gee, you've lost a few pounds!" can create temporary feelings of self-esteem, but there are often negative consequences as well. In their dieting efforts many young women begin to harbor obsessive, selfish, and competitive feelings toward other women, gloating secretly when others are overweight. While they may want friendship, their preoccupation with body and their shyness keeps them from gaining friends (or from being a good friend themselves).

The way the adolescent girl deals with the disillusionment and unfulfilled expectations about weight can be crucial. The follow-

ing account casts light on how the feelings of despair and emptiness following dieting attempts can facilitate bulimarexic behavior:
"I guess I started feeling down about myself and my weight in
seventh grade. I was about five feet tall and weighed 120 pounds.
Since no boy would want to 'go out' with Minnesota Fats (one of
my nicknames), I became the matchmaker for everyone. I was the
one a boy would call up if he liked one of my friends. I was also the
one who would be called if someone needed a homework assignment. Furthermore, I was the one who helped plan the dances and
then spent the night sitting on the garbage can in the girl's locker
room. I played the part of the class clown, thinking that if I made
people laugh they wouldn't care if I was fat. Finally, at the end of
ninth grade, I decided to do something about my weight. I lost 10
pounds and grew two inches. . . ."

This young woman goes on to describe the anger and confusion
she felt upon discovering that her weight loss brought her no
greater social success. She returned to being "social chairman" and
"good ole girl" and slowly gained back all her weight and then
some. Soon after, she initiated the binge/purge cycle that was to
cripple her life for thirteen years. Such unrealistic and unfulfilled
expectations about weight are crucial in the subsequent development of both anorexia and bulimarexia. The bulimarexic embarks
on a Harlequin existence, hiding her pain and loneliness and living in dread that her "disgusting" habit will be exposed. She is not
retreating from the challenges and responsibilities of being a
woman, as the anorexic is, but is trying too hard to conform to the
feminine ideal.

If she manages to survive the agony of these adolescent years,
there is another traumatic period that may very well propel her toward one or the other of these eating disorders. This is the period
when she makes the important break from her family, home, community, and school and enters college or begins a career.

5.

The College Years and Beyond

In 1946 Mirra Komarovsky, a sociologist, surveyed female students at Barnard College in order to assess the various academic and social pressures they were experiencing. Many of these young women admitted to being confused about conflicting expectations from family and other relatives. One student stated her dilemma as follows: "Uncle John telephones every Sunday morning. His first question is: 'Did you go out last night?' He would think me a grind if I were to stay home Saturday night to finish a term paper. My father expects me to get an A in every subject and is disappointed by a B. He says I have plenty of time for a social life. Mother says that 'A in Philosophy is very nice dear, but please don't become so deep that no man will be good enough for you.' " Komarovsky's studies were conducted over forty years ago. Optimistically, we would imagine that the impact of the women's liberation movement has eliminated more traditional standards of feminine behavior and encouraged independent achievement for women. However, if Komarovsky had visited a college campus today and polled its female students, she would have been surprised to find responses almost identical to those of her 1946 survey. The paradoxical messages from family and society as a whole have continued with distressing persistence. On the one hand, the young women are expected to excel academically, to be attractive, and to have an active social life; on the other, they are encouraged to remain "invisible," which translates to mean not too self-reliant, assertive, or serious.

The middle-class bulimarexic women who began to fill our therapy groups appeared even more protected, helpless, and desperate for male approval than their 1946 counterparts. In addition, they were overwhelmed by concerns about physical appearance and the pursuit of slimness. Joanne, one of our initial Cornell group members, articulated these traditional and contemporary concerns during her first interview: "I feel my body is ugly and I'm not really worthwhile! I realize I feel that most acutely after I speak to my parents. My father wants to know how the grades are. My mother asks, each time she calls, if I have put on weight. If I say yes, she tells me I won't be able to attract a man. Deep down inside I don't want to turn my back on my parents because I believe being skinny, an A student, and attracting a man with a desirable career will satisfy their demands as well as my own."

Many women who survive their adolescent years without disordered responses to food seem especially vulnerable during their early years at college. New opportunities present themselves, and new pressures move in. The experience of being a freshman, in somewhat threatening and unfamiliar surroundings, can be a traumatic one for even the most well adjusted young adult. The overprotected women we were seeing felt the separation from family most acutely. On their own for the first time in their lives, confronted by new people and possibilities, and away from the mealtime routines of the days when they lived at home, women who had never had weight problems began to put on pounds. Often family members reacted more negatively to the rapid weight gain than did the women themselves. One woman, who initially had satisfactory social experiences, had this to say:

Once in college I met guys right away and began to enjoy dating, and even kissing and making out as long as we didn't "go too far." Dates involved eating out a great deal—pizza and beer usually—and I returned home from this first year of college happy but 20 pounds heavier. At 5'2" and 125 pounds, I was pleasingly plump, but not to my mother, who was horrified with the changes in my body. My frequent snacking was looked on with disgust, so I was happy to return to college in the fall, away from my mother's disapproving eye.

When this young woman returned to college, she, like many others, shifted her dependency from family to the college itself. Campus life, although frightening, provided a certain structure and protection and a hope for the future. The women came to view college as their big chance (some viewed it as their last chance), and their definition of success was rigid and extreme: they must receive straight A's and they must be pursued by men. If they received lower marks than those to which they were accustomed, they felt despair. If they were not socially active and did not form intimate relationships with men, they considered themselves worthless and incomplete.

With such expectations, they set themselves up for failure. In the seventies, campuses had lost the freewheeling sense of camaraderie fostered by the political activism and defiance of the sixties. The academic atmosphere was more serious and good grades harder to maintain. Noses were to the grindstone, competition was fierce, and students felt more isolated and lonely. The women's movement had made some inroads, but even if some women had acquired a new consciousness, it was clear that many more defined themselves in terms of male approval. If they were not sought after by men, they were failures.

The women we were seeing had a long history of perfectionism, and they were of above-average intelligence. For the most part, they had done well at school and felt somewhat secure in this area (although they were quick to characterize themselves as social failures). Thus, an increased push toward academic achievement quickly became their way of compensating for feelings of social inadequacy and self-doubt—especially if male attention was not immediately forthcoming. Eventually, however, even academic success failed to counter the emptiness they experienced when their expectations of being pursued by men did not materialize. As we have seen, the majority of these women had been both desirous of and frightened by male contact during adolescence. Now, feeling an intense urgency to form intimate relationships, they believed themselves unattractive, undesirable, and unworthy, and many turned to food for solace.

Some women spoke of food as an "inadequate means of coping, a return to old childhood security." For others, eating became a form of entertainment. "I was eating alone for the first time in my life." The change in eating habits was often bolstered by the fact that "others were in the same boat." One of our freshman coeds said: "The first eating bout that could be classified as a binge was during a period of loneliness when I felt overwhelmed by the size of Cornell. Heterosexual relationships were nil at this point and the only pressure I felt to be thin was the sign of thin girls and dieting friends."

During their college years, other women turn away from food and toward "The Diet" in hopes of finding the key to social success. When their expectations for a magical transformation are not realized, they, like their adolescent counterparts, often begin to binge after one or several dieting attempts have failed. Initially, as in the following example, they may not have been overweight, but they then allow themselves to become a slave to the habit: "At the beginning of my freshman year of college, I decided that at 128 pounds and 5′6″, I was fat. I began a crash diet and lost 15 pounds. During the next summer I lived away from home by myself and literally ate myself into 160 pounds of ugliness out of loneliness. I began to purge out of total desperation soon after."

Overwhelmed by the pressures and demands of college, a woman may decide to lose a little weight and then become obsessed and intoxicated with the weight loss. Disturbed emotional, cognitive, and behavioral patterns emerge from the assault and stress of food deprivation. The same self-perpetuating mechanisms occur. Dieting has become what Judith Rodin, a Yale psychologist, calls a "normative obsession." Often the weight loss leads to compliments and feelings of triumph. The problems with school now are replaced with a problem of how to lose more weight. However, suddenly there is no rhyme or reason to the weight loss, and the original "ideal" number no longer seems good enough. As they continue to lose weight, body image disparagement and body image perception of "fat" intensifies. Losing weight succeeds in becoming a major accomplishment and may provide a temporary respite from the stress that led to a decision to diet. So whether by accident or intent, the end result is the same: Anorexia still starts to run the show.

Thus dieting characterized by extreme denial leads to anorexia or often binges that may continue for months.

During the summer between my freshman and sophomore years of college, I lost 35 pounds and continued to diet through Thanksgiving, being very proud of the fact that I made it through a Thanksgiving dinner with the family without cheating. Actually, in five months I had never once deviated from the diet I was following, never had even one bite of "illegal" food. I came back to school after the holiday and went to dinner with some friends. I suddenly decided to have a piece of chocolate cream pie. Once I ate this, I felt there was nothing stopping me. I felt singularly directed—I had to have another "bad" thing to eat. I went immediately to the store and bought a bag of cookies; next I had some ice cream and on and on. This binge didn't let up until February. Never once did I feel I had control over this process. I blamed the binge, the weight gain, my depression, *everything,* on that one piece of pie. I said over and over, "If only I hadn't eaten the pie." It was as though I had an ultimately fatal disease—although there were periods of remission, it was certainly a terminal case with no real hope of recovery.

Some women do experience moderate social success, but not enough to give them the necessary confidence. Even while they are dating, a chance remark about weight by a man can precipitate the destructive eating pattern. Ellen traces her problem to such an experience: "Early in my sophomore year I met Peter, my future husband. He told me, practically on our first date, that if I lost a little weight I'd be beautiful. I began dieting strenuously at that point and lost 25 pounds. I soon became compulsive about keeping my weight at 98 throughout my college years and did so by replacing pizza and beer with yogurt, grapefruit, and black coffee." Although Ellen was able to maintain her "ideal" weight throughout college, she gained a few pounds when she was in graduate school. She tried a number of dieting methods without success and then remembered that a college roommate with a similar problem had forced herself to vomit. Ellen was so unhappy with her weight gain that she tried this method. It seemed to work, so she began an eight-year pattern of bingeing and purging.

Those women who have already initiated a binge/purge cycle in adolescence face additional obstacles to intimacy with men once they enter college. The binge/purge cycle of bulimarexics is so confining that an inordinate amount of energy is expended simply in the behavior, and the women are unable to concentrate on anything else. Paradoxically, these women who yearn so intensely for intimacy report feeling most vulnerable when they are with men. They are then at their most isolated, living in a way that is basically dishonest, and convinced that they must hide their inner selves from the world. They live in dread that their eating habits will be exposed and that men will reject them. Most of these women have had limited dating experience and therefore lack confidence in social situations.

Many of the women we treated had never had a lasting or loving relationship with a man. They hoped therapy would help them change in ways that would "turn guys on." Success was defined as losing more weight and staying that way. Lacking any insight into their problem, they could not (would not) feel "whole" without a man. If only "Prince Charming" would appear, everything would be all right. At the same time, they were unable to see how their neediness and desperation drove men to reject them. These women have great difficulty viewing themselves as capable of developing into strong and independent women. In their encounters with men, they are constantly trying to find out what the man likes. If he is a tennis player, they take up tennis. If classical music is his interest, they follow that pursuit with a vengeance. A woman named Stephanie told us: "I knocked myself out doing things that were against my nature. All for the purpose of making him notice me. The relationship ended after a few months. My problems in concentration started soon after. He used to be my motivation all through school, and then he dropped me away. Schoolwork became meaningless. If I could have anything or anybody, I would still want him. I have a feeling only another man can take my mind off this preoccupation."

Another woman said: "I've been guiding my life toward my Prince Charming, and it's probably not going to happen. That's pretty scary."

Recently, we addressed the student body of a small eastern college about our research and treatment of bulimarexia. During the question-and-answer period, a coed mentioned a letter to the editor of their campus newspaper that had created a furor. The facts were a bit fuzzy, but evidently a male student had written to say that the women students of the college had "let themselves go" physically. He described them as having "fat asses." The coed cited the letter as an example of the ways men put women under pressure. During her presentation, Marlene had indicated that in spite of the so-called new feminism, the present model of extreme slimness was being imposed *on women by women*—i.e., men do not prefer Twiggys or Kate Mosses! This woman was saying no to Marlene and using the letter to show that men expected extreme thinness in women. After the letter appeared in the newspaper, widespread dieting among the women resulted, and some began to dread eating in the dining centers. Not only were they convinced that male students were watching them eat, but they began to watch each other eat as well. As this woman was telling her story, we noticed many other women nodding in agreement. What was most significant and striking to us were the women's own reactions to the opinion of *one* man. Rather than ignoring the letter or responding with humor (even anger), these women believed themselves unattractive and, by extension, incapable of attracting men.

The ability to reward herself, to feel her own self-worth, is foreign to the bulimarexic, who seems intent on pleasing others and being perfect. Ironically, her very behavior serves to keep her socially isolated. Anne's story provides a fairly typical example. For months, Anne had been secretly fasting and bingeing. Then she was invited out to dinner by a young man with whom she was infatuated. She wanted to accept the date but was in the fasting part of her cycle. She was afraid that she would give in to temptation and eat and thus worked herself into a high state of anxiety. Should she go on the date or stay at home? She did accept, ate moderately at dinner, and had an enjoyable time. But after the man had seen her home, the stress of the evening proved to be too much for her, and she began to binge grotesquely. The disgust that followed her binge provided Anne with an excuse to withdraw from further social encounters.

Many women like Anne are so frightened by the possibility of rejection that it seems safer to hide behind fat or disgust than to risk actual engagement. Because of their low self-esteem, these women feel unworthy of being loved and can attribute this feeling to their temporary self-disgust about bingeing or being slightly overweight. Bingeing wards off people with a "wall of (perceived) fat." It is a way of "filling up" without needing others.

The woman so afflicted becomes locked into a struggle between two parts of herself. Total control versus being out of control—being "good" versus being "bad." The bulimarexic, believing herself unlovable, then becomes supersensitive to the reactions of others. The most minor or insignificant slight is exaggerated and distorted, creating massive self-loathing that propels the woman to further bingeing. The anger she feels toward her imagined rejector is not acknowledged. Instead, it is turned inward, adding to the fury of the binge.

The insidious fear of rejection often evolves into irrational and crippling thoughts. These naïve and unassertive women focus on rejection alone, rather than on the man who has rejected them. They rarely examine his human failings, nor can they conceive of themselves as fortunate to be rid of someone who does not value them. There is a life-and-death quality to these relationships even when it is clear that the women are only marginally involved. It does not seem to matter if they do not even *like* the man who has rejected them or if the man has obviously been using and/or abusing them. Being rejected therefore is equated with being a failure. Significantly, most lack the courage to ask their partners about what went wrong. They weave a rich fantasy around the experience, assuming the worst—that they have been rejected because they are too fat!

Some bulimarexic women do develop intimate relationships with men. This can lead to a "remission" of symptoms (as long as these caring men are in the picture). Once involved with a man, however, they typically rechannel most of the energy they have been expending on bingeing and purging into a mutually destructive/dependent relationship. Aimee Liu, the author of *Solitaire,* appears deliberately to have made this trade-off when she chose to apply to the same college her boyfriend was attending: "It suddenly occurred to me that love might help me escape the tyranny of my eating compulsions, that in fact those compulsions were probably offshoots of loneliness and insecurity. All the stuffing and subsequent self-abuse had helped to pass time that should have been devoted to someone else. But now that Ken was ready to save me, I could normalize."

Rather than residing in a college dorm, Aimee moved in with her boyfriend and did in fact normalize her eating behavior. However, she soon found that she had become an extension of Ken. Eventually, she had to break this dependency before she could grow as a healthy and self-actualized woman.

Such relationships, while relieving the surface of the bulimarexic's problem, are generally ultimately destructive. The neediness of these women makes the possibility of success uncertain, and termination of the affair is experienced as devastating—driving the woman even deeper into hopelessness and helplessness, and increasing her anger toward men.

Some, while in the throes of such relationships, resume their bingeing, thereby resorting to dishonesty and subterfuge. Even if they are competent in all other aspects of their lives, they do not feel whole, functioning, or "normal." They live in fear that they will be "found out." Since these women have invested their men with heroic qualities, they can only experience themselves as smaller and weaker by comparison. Believing themselves so unworthy, they are grateful that women as "screwed up" and disgusting as themselves could be lucky enough to find men who love them. Since they also believe that their men "love a lie," they necessarily experience themselves as "phony" and unreal.

Heterosexual relationships then are a parody—an exaggeration of all that is wrong with these women's lives. However powerless and helpless they may feel in relation to school or family, they are even more debilitated when involved in relationships that are sexual. Sexuality is a great wasteland of unfulfilled pleasures, confusion, guilt, fear, and disgust. Many are protected and relatively innocent women who have generally been brought up to be "good girls." Promiscuity, liberal or carefree sexual attitudes, and multiple sexual relationships are conspicuously absent from their lives. The following is a typical comment: "I have always been very naïve about sexual relationships. I can remember pondering whether it was a sin when someone touched my breast for the first time when I was nineteen! I was shocked to learn that my roommate had been sleeping with her boyfriend since she was sixteen."

Our research suggests that sex and sexual fantasies play an important part in the lives of these women. Here we are not referring to the fantasy of oral impregnation that appears in much of the analytic literature about women with eating disorders but to the fear of rejection by the sexual partner. In other words, the woman is afraid she is not good enough to please a man. Bulimarexics are, of course, not alone in these fears. Most women have been conditioned to accept men as more experienced sexually and to expect them to be the teachers in sexual matters.

In addition, the lifetime socialization of women trains them to derive their pleasure from *giving* rather from receiving. Until recently, the standards for appropriate sexual behavior have been set for women by men. Women should be supremely sensitive to the needs of the men they are involved with, always concerned that the men be satisfied. This preoccupation with pleasing men leads women to lose connection with their own desires and needs. Many bulimarexic women unquestioningly accept their partners' idea of what sexual activity is acceptable. When the women do not achieve satisfaction, they blame themselves, feel that they are failures. It sel-

dom occurs to them to expect pleasure for its own sake (their pleasure is in giving), nor are they assertive enough or candid enough
to indicate the kind of touching they find pleasurable. Thus, while
many of these women are sexually active, they do not experience
fulfillment. They feel they must go through whatever charade is
necessary to secure the love and attention of their men. Some fake
orgasm, while others seek to avoid sexual intercourse, though they
may find kissing and caressing pleasurable, because they feel that
intercourse leaves them vulnerable to rejection if their performance
should not be considered satisfactory. Being a good sex partner is
equated with being a "real woman."

Sometimes the fear of sexuality takes a different form. There are
women who are afraid that their appetite for sex will become as insatiable as their appetite for food. Since they overwhelmingly feel
out of control with regard to food, they come to feel that they are
powerless over their sexual behavior as well. Consequently, they
binge on sex on occasion and punish themselves with the same feelings of shame and self-disgust that they use against themselves
after food orgies. Not surprisingly, such empty and dehumanizing
sexual encounters often create a further stimulus for grotesque
food binges. "I habitually use food as an insulator," one woman
told us. "It protects me from sexual contact and promiscuity. When
I am thin, I become sexual, constantly worrying about sexual performance and wondering if I will be able to have an orgasm this
time. Wondering if the man will know I feign it. Ironically, the
men with whom I sleep invariably shower me with praise for my
skill as a lover. Afterward I try to relieve my insecurity with food.
After a man leaves my apartment, I rush to the mirror to see if yet
another sexual encounter has changed me. It hasn't, so I will devote
an entire day to bingeing."

Along with the fear of being an inadequate sexual partner, bulimarexics typically loathe their bodies. They are certain that they
will be rejected because they are too fat, and they believe that men
will be horrified to see them undressed. If they do appear naked,
they are likely to require constant reassurance that their bodies are
attractive. Many allow themselves to sleep only in one position

(on their stomachs), for fear that their lovers will see a protruding stomach. Such narcissistic self-absorption can cause their worst fears to come true. The lover who is badgered incessantly by the woman who asks if he thinks she's too fat is bound eventually to respond with anger or boredom.

Although recent research has indicated that men are more attracted to women's faces than to their bodies, bulimarexics think they already know what men really want. They are absolutely convinced that their bodies are imperfect; therefore, it is irrelevant what their men say to them.

Undoubtedly, Jackie, the woman whose story follows, would like to be thought of as a sharp lady who is exciting to be with, but her preoccupation with appearance has narrowed her to the point where she is no longer stimulating or interesting. She may feel a perverse satisfaction that her lover has confirmed her deepest fears, and she may not realize that she is the one who is driving him away. Jackie and women like her turn themselves into sexual objects, albeit unwittingly. Often, the men with whom they have relationships want women who are quite different from the image the bulimarexics hold in mind. This man Jackie's fiancé, at his wit's end, wrote the following:

Lately, all our conversations center around Jackie's body. She used to be witty, fun, and exciting. I was attracted to her enthusiasm and her mind. She was and still is (although I'm beginning to doubt this) a very sharp lady. However, she now sounds like a broken record. After we finish talking about her body she has nothing to say. I could care less if she's ten to fifteen pounds heavier and that is the God's honest truth! In fact, I would prefer it, as right now she looks like a refugee! Of course, though, she doesn't believe me. She insists she knows *what I really like*—even what I am thinking. I find this infuriating.

Few bulimarexics report that they started bingeing and purging while married, although several turn to this form of solace when separated or divorced. Many, however, vow to give up gorging and purging once they are married. The hope is that marriage itself will magically transform their lives. For some this does happen, and they experience long remissions. Others resume their habit in secret, feeling more guilty and ashamed than ever. And with good reason, for their lives are filled with further subterfuge. Now, in addition to bingeing and purging, the woman depletes her energy with games she must invent to cover her tracks. She has little time for anything other than nurturing the behavior, engaging in it, and hiding it. Honesty, intimacy, and mutual respect become impossible under such circumstances. When these marriages fail, the men may never really know what happened. Unbelievable as it may seem, bulimarexics have managed to keep their behavior a total secret from husbands and other loved ones for as long as ten to fifteen years. Upon observing their wives' exaggerated sense of privacy, some husbands suspect the worst: "She must be having an affair," they conclude. If their wives do reveal a "problem with food," these husbands are vastly relieved; a food problem seems insignificant when compared to what they had fantasized. Other husbands are bewildered by what they see as abuse of the body. From boyhood, they have been taught to "build up" and conserve their bodies, not to tear them down, and they have always viewed themselves as *much more* than their bodies alone. As Susan Sontag pointed out in her article "The Double Standard of Aging," men traditionally have been conditioned to feel that it is not masculine to care so much about their looks (while women are conditioned "to care too much"). Thus, many men, no matter how sympathetic they might be, find the excessive vanity of bulimarexics ludicrous, frivolous, foolish, and downright boring. They honestly cannot comprehend that women could make themselves slaves to food. In their confusion, they deny that there is a problem and somehow believe that if they ignore it, it will go away. When wives finally reach out for help from these men, the response is often totally unexpected: "His reaction was very similar to what many people had said to me. Psychiatrists, for instance. What I told him went in one ear and out the other. I couldn't convey the intensity of my problem to him. My food binges didn't seem like a serious thing—he thought I was ridiculous."

One woman who had maintained bulimarexia throughout twelve years of marriage finally chose her thirteenth wedding anniversary as the time to "confess." Her husband responded with a burst of laughter and refused to listen to her further attempts to explain. In so doing, he was giving her an all clear to continue the binge/purge behavior because the message implicit in his reaction was "It's not so serious" or "It's OK for you to do this screwy thing." In this case, revealing the secret created further conflict as communication was still blocked. Husbands can also use the confession as leverage with their wives, controlling them through threats of exposure or rejection. Furthermore, with this new ammunition they can retaliate if their wives dare to criticize them for their own imperfections.

Other husbands become suspicious and angry. Not knowing what course to take, they adopt a watchdog stance, which often makes matters worse. One despairing husband put it this way: "This problem controls her whole schedule and dictates that much time be devoted to her problem. She cheats both herself and me out of time. I feel she lies to 'cover' her secret behavior. She locks bathroom doors so she can engage in her habit in privacy, and then I start assuming she's engaging in bingeing or more likely vomiting, especially when this occurs after I go to bed."

Husbands who refuse to take bulimarexia seriously are not necessarily insensitive or uncaring. Some are initially understanding, but when the behavior does not lessen, they reach their limits. Typically, they say they do not care if their wives are slightly overweight—they just want them to be happy again, the way they were at some earlier time. Afraid for the future, these men are actually trying to encourage their wives to be stronger and less dependent. Intuitively, they feel that they are lending support to the behavior if they monitor their wives or become too involved in their care. They want to see their wives take more responsibility for their own actions, to see them be *partners* in the truest sense, and they are motivated by love and an understanding of contemporary psychology. The dangerous nature of too much involvement is clearly illustrated by a conversation we had with a demoralized husband a few years ago. This man called one evening and insisted on speaking to Bill. In desperation, he wanted to know if he was doing the right thing. For the last few months, his wife had asked him to assist her in throwing up after bingeing by standing behind her and pulling on her stomach. She said she could not vomit by herself. This man loved his wife but obviously felt deeply uncertain about her request. Bill simply asked him how he felt about *his* participation in the ritual. Apparently, the man had seldom been asked about *his* feelings. He said he was disgusted by what he was doing. In fact, he knew that his wife's binges had increased since he took on the role of accomplice. Bill told him that it was appropriate for him to feel such revulsion, and this seemed to help. The man told his wife that he honestly felt she was killing herself and their relationship and that he could not aid and abet her any longer. He insisted that she seek treatment immediately. After some resistance, she did.

What is going wrong in these marriages? For the most part, bulimarexics trade their individual talents and outside activities for the romantic ideal of security, safety, and living happily ever after with their husbands. Eagerly discarding career objectives in order to devote themselves to the wife-homemaker role, they now have feelings of "entitlement." In return, they should be rescued from responsibility and cared for. However, *vicarious* living is especially difficult for bulimarexics since before marriage they were generally high achievers. The burden for bulimarexics is their *history*. Most, at one point or another, have been rewarded for their accomplishments and have experienced the exhilaration of using their talents. It is an experience they yearn for again and again, even though they have locked themselves into a limited role.

Current research indicates that level of education is an important variable in marriage satisfaction. According to many surveys, college educated women are consistently less satisfied with the homemaker role than those without such an education. With fewer sources of outside gratification available, they soon become bored, depressed, and unhappy. In time, a husband's successes coupled with the wife's increasing emptiness and envy often signify the death of a marriage. Shirley, college educated and a talented musician, is a good example. Her family and friends were overjoyed when she met, "captured," and married Sam, a well-known surgeon. Sad to say, her own years of accomplishment as a concert pianist had never elicited as much acceptance and excitement. After three years of comparative idleness, Shirley, feeling herself an extension of Sam, began to have minor but unpredictable temper tantrums. In reaction, Sam began to spend more and more time at the hospital. Shirley, in a panic at losing Sam, alternated between "perfect wife" tactics and withdrawal. Since Shirley had given up bulimarexia "forever" on the day she married, this obviously was not her problem *now.* However, she almost wished it were because she was unable, even with the help of intensive psychotherapy, to understand what her real conflicts were. She believed, and therapy reinforced the belief, that she had everything she had ever dreamed of. So what was wrong with her. Why couldn't she relax and be nice, appreciative, and grateful? What Shirley thought she "should" feel prevented her from ever facing up to her lack of fulfillment in a direct fashion. In part, this was not Shirley's fault. Like many women, she had chosen a man whose credentials were "perfect." By comparison, Shirley felt inadequate and insignificant, and since she had abandoned her concert career without a backward glance, it was hard for Sam to take her talent seriously. She, in turn, reinforced this by "playing for Sam" (i.e., popular music), thus giving up playing what she loved most—Beethoven and Bach. Eventually, Sam grew tired of Shirley's instability and nagging and walked out. On that day she resumed the old familiar habit she had given up four years before—bingeing and purging.

Colette Dowling, in *The Cinderella Complex: Women's Hidden Fear of Independence,* captures some of the dynamics of bulimarexic women when she describes the way in which married women embrace drudge work to preserve their illusion of security and to avoid challenging responsibilities as well as their terror of aloneness and the unknown. Dowling's book is about the ways women themselves contribute to their own states of helplessness and nurture the desire to merge with another person. The book is provocative because Dowling exposes the ways women manipulate and exploit men in order to get them to take care of them so that they can lead childlike, easy, and unchallenged lives.

In our group therapy program, many married bulimarexic women have concluded that this behavior is characteristic of them. By relinquishing responsibility and embracing the role of the "sick one," the bulimarexic creates further conflicts for her husband as well as for herself. Anne's husband, Paul, a concerned and loving man, felt at least partially responsible for her unhappiness. She felt he loved his work more than her, and Paul, out of a genuine desire to help Anne through her "crisis," began to spend more time at home. Anne had literally taken to bed after being laid off from a high status job. The state of the economy rather than poor performance had resulted in the layoff, but Anne had chosen to do nothing and had become very depressed. She returned to a childhood pattern of overeating, gained fifteen pounds in only six weeks, and then refused to go out. Although she had often gained weight and then fasted during similar stress periods while in college, she had triumphantly stabilized her eating habits for the two years of her marriage. As his worries increased, Paul began giving up those physical activities he used to let off steam after a grueling day as a salesman. He stopped playing squash with his buddies and gave up his greatest love—fly-fishing in the wilderness. His role as caretaker for Anne only seemed to make matters worse. When he complied with Anne's requests to keep her from eating by locking cabinets, she became angry, even defiant, and accused him of not really wanting to be with her. In fact, her accusation was starting to become a reality. She was becoming harder and harder to love. Paul felt he was "the man," the one who should be able to solve the problem. However, lately he had been feeling more and more ineffectual.

Numerous concerned men have shared similar feelings of despair and frustration over "losing their wives," women who have obviously expected more from them than any one person could provide. The pain and victimization of these men is as intense as that of their partners.

Of course, there are husbands whose personal problems are overwhelming. Many bulimarexics simply have terrible marital relationships that can hardly be considered the end result of bulimarexia, although it might be said that their fantasies of rescue kept them from seeing men clearly in the first place. Whether the men are alcoholic, irresponsible, self-occupied, or downright hostile and abusive, a terrifying fear of being alone combined with a paralyzing sense of guilt and helplessness keeps the women imprisoned in destructive relationships with them. Most of these women have been conditioned to believe it is up to them to make the marriage work, even when there is no longer anything to be retrieved. There must be something they are doing wrong or should be doing right. They suffer all kinds of abuse as the price for holding onto the illusion that things will get better if they just try harder, or love more, or seek therapy. For these desperately unhappy women, gorging and purging can become a crucial coping mechanism. Their marriages will continue to be terrible whether or not they give up the behavior. Bingeing and purging serves to keep the painful reality of their lives temporarily buried. Instead of making a decision—in short, taking action—they prefer treading water, avoiding, and hoping.

Some bulimarexic women do attempt to break away from mutually destructive marriages. Unfortunately, many act impulsively. They may abruptly move out of the house, hoping that they will be able to give up bulimarexia. After all, most continue to believe that bulimarexia is their real problem, not their husbands or their marriages. If they can just resolve their food problem everything will be OK! But now they are alone with their food. Almost invariably, they crash and return home to their husbands. Those who manage to make the break from their marital relationships generally transfer their dependency needs back to families, friends, or therapists. With few supports available, they are unable to move forward on their own. In a particularly poignant letter, one woman stated: "I had reached the point where I was having trouble coping with day-to-day activities. I couldn't get out of bed and go to work. I was really in bad shape, and I wasn't able to confide in my husband, get help from him. I didn't have any friends where we were. I called my family out of desperation, not knowing what to do. I just cried . . . didn't really tell them what was going on. Just told them everything was terrible, and my father said, 'Come home. We'll take care of you. We'll make everything better.' " And so this woman traded one kind of dependency for another, more benign, form.

What if there are children? Does the prospect of caring for another human being who is even more helpless and dependent cause a change in behavior? Once again, the expectations of many bulimarexic women are unrealistic. There is always the hope that an outside situation will release them magically from their disordered eating behavior. And, in most cases, they experience disappointment. As one women told us: "I can recall only one week of abstinence after my pregnancy. I was afraid that vomiting would tear my stitches. You see, even the fear that I might hurt my unborn child would not make me stop this habit."

Bulimarexic women who continue their behavior throughout pregnancy and the rearing of children often seem more helpless and desperate than their married, childless counterparts. For, in addition to feelings of shame and self-disgust, they carry the added burden of believing that they are bad mothers. Their guilt is often overwhelming.

Many mothers report that they looked forward to childbirth, believing their eating compulsion would be replaced with new goals and self-fulfilling activities. In addition to child care, some become compulsive house cleaners or harness their own compulsion to eat by becoming gourmet cooks for others—children, husbands, and friends. They throw themselves into a frenzy of activity that makes them seem the perfect mother and wife. More than likely, however, these women resume their habitual bingeing patterns: "I don't want to die, but I am killing myself. I have two children, and yet my obsession with food comes first. I work and cook a decent meal for my children every night, which I don't eat. I wait until they are through, eat everything they haven't, which is usually a lot, and then eat everything else I can find, usually sweet. I am a good mother, *I guess,* but I hate myself."

Still living through others, they are essentially the same passive, dependent, and nonassertive women they were at the time they married. While family responsibilities and society's expectations have broadened and become more complex, their inner selves are still embryonic, fuzzy, and undefined.

Bulimarexic wives and mothers often point wistfully to the unmarried career women in our groups. Most are amazed that these supposedly independent women also feel dissatisfaction and emptiness. They find it confusing, for our therapy emphasizes the need for more than one identity and for taking action and risks. Here are these attractive and talented women, out in the world and growing through their success. But are they? The fact is that more than a few of these professional women envy the married woman. They would gladly set aside the anxiety involved in daily risk taking and confrontation for the comfort and security they believe is inherent in marriage and childbearing. Some even express resentment that they *have* to support themselves. Unlike married bulimarexics, single career women do not usually binge out of boredom. On the contrary, their lives are often *too* full, and as perpetual people pleasers they habitually take on more than they can handle. Their bingeing is often precipitated because of their unwillingness to say no and give themselves a break. Becoming a career woman does not signal the death of the "good girl." In spite of their achievements, many still have great difficulty dealing with disapproval and criticism. Besides, now that they have proven their success to all, there is constant pressure to continue doing so. Thus it is not surprising that few of our professional women are comfortable with the power associated with the work world or with the excellence that is now expected of them.

Of course, we have encountered professional women who do gain real satisfaction from their careers and they have every intention of continuing to work, whether or not they become wives and mothers. Their hope is that they will be able to combine all the roles. Their problem lies not in career overinvolvement but in social underinvolvement. They may have professional strengths, but they are still shy and nonassertive with men. They long for relationships but lack confidence and social skills. In one very important way, they are similar to married bulimarexics—they continue to value the importance of relationships with men above all else and to give men the power to define how they should act, think, and feel.

6.

Eating Disorders and the Body

As we pointed out in the first edition of this book, our aim in this chapter is not to scare women out of bingeing and purging. Scare tactics are seldom successful in convincing people to change habits. However, we do want to make women aware of the damage they may be inflicting on their bodies. The factual material presented here is an update of recent research and includes what we have learned from medical colleagues and the literature. We continue to draw extensively on what we have learned from clients—particularly clients who are physicians, nurses, and nutritionists. We are particularly indebted to Bruce L. Fariss, M.D., our endocrinology consultant, and to Pat Young, our nutritional consultant, for their help in updating this important chapter.

If after reading this chapter some women are persuaded to modify their eating behavior, we will be enormously pleased. More women are now confiding in their physicians directly and candidly about all aspects of their problem, as evidenced by the calls and letters we continue to receive from doctors. Such professionals also publish and meet regularly to discuss their patients, thereby educating the community. Despite these encouraging changes, we hope that by focusing attention on this major threat to women's health, we can encourage professionals to question and examine their patients more thoroughly. For, as we have stressed repeatedly, covert pleas for help are often overlooked or misinterpreted.

THE BINGE

Binge eating is well recognized as a problem among people of all weight levels. Independent research at Duke and Stanford universities has indicated that approximately 50 percent of the obese patients surveyed binged on large quantities of food at least once a week. Our survey data with regard to bulimarexics is even more dramatic. Of three hundred polled, 82 percent indicated that they binged at least three times a week.

Bingers tend to prefer high-calorie junk food, although they will binge on anything that is readily available. Fast foods high in sugar content that require little preparation are prime binge foods, particularly when they can be quickly purchased and consumed in private. Here are some of the problems that can result.

Hypoglycemia

Many bulimarexics attribute their dizziness, headaches, fatigue, numbness, irritability, crying, excessive worry, anxiety, and depression to a syndrome known as hypoglycemia. Hypoglycemia literally refers to a deficiency of sugar in the blood. Although it is at the opposite pole from diabetes, it can often be the first manifestation of a tendency toward that disease. In hypoglycemia, the body, in response to foods high in sugar content, triggers the pancreas to release an excess of insulin. Repeated bingeing (which tends to amplify this excessive insulin response to carbohydrates in a person predisposed to diabetes because of a family history of that disease) drives blood-sugar levels below normal, often creating a craving for more sugar—the very substance that initiated the disorder in the first place. Thus, hypoglycemics often turn to foods that are forbidden in order to satisfy this "craving." Examples of these forbidden foods are sugar, honey, pizza, breads made from refined flour, potatoes, corn, rice, and sugar-sweetened soft drinks.

Recently, researchers more attuned to the binge/purge practices of thousands of women began to question this "craving for sugar" excuse of the bulimarexic. Dr. L. M. Vincent, writing in *Competing with the Sylph,* feels that the incidence of true chemical hypoglycemia has been exaggerated, often serving as a convenient scapegoat for those women who fail to acknowledge or are unaware of the harm they are causing their bodies by gorging and purging. Dr. Vincent indicates that a combination of psychological and physiological factors contributes to the desire to binge; i.e., severe carbohydrate restriction could lead to carbohydrate craving. Under such circumstances, it is dangerous for the chronic binger to hide behind the hypoglycemic label, for in doing so she not only finds an excuse for her inability to maintain proper nutrition but stubbornly refuses to explore alternative sources of her problem. She has a disease, and, as with all good patients, she must be cured—by someone else!

Dr. Vincent therefore emphasizes the importance of distinguishing "pseudohypoglycemia," which can be traced to the poor nutritional status of the binge/purger, from true chemical hypoglycemia.

Anecdotal evidence gleaned from the bulimarexics we have treated supports the view that poor diet and stress initiate the fatigue, dizziness, and anxiety associated with pseudohypoglycemia. These symptoms are usually reversible within a few months, and bulimarexics who embark on appropriate corrective nutritional programs report that their internists soon consider them healthy again. However, in *every* case initiation and maintenance of this supplementary medical treatment was related to the women's willingness to enter psychotherapy and honestly confront the problem on more than one level. For this reason we have developed a network of informed internists, endocrinologists, and nutritionists who are prepared to help the eating-disorder clients who are determined to help themselves. Such an interdisciplinary approach should be an integral part of any comprehensive treatment program.

Metabolic Considerations

Bulimarexics apparently do not realize that fat synthesis and accumulation are necessary for survival. Fat is the main storage form of body energy, although sugar, stored in our muscles, is our most immediately available source. However, sugar is in limited supply, and when it is depleted, fatigue and exhaustion ultimately occur. Thus under the usual demands of our daily routine, we draw upon fatty acids (fats) as a major source of energy. In fact, doctors tell us that with mild exercise, fat contributes twice as much energy as does sugar. However, when fat levels are depleted, the body must draw upon carbohydrates (sugar). The blood-sugar level is therefore critical and is indirectly regulated by the pancreas, which releases insulin according to body needs when we are hungry, as after exercise. Sugar supplies dwindle so that insulin inhibition stimulates the release of more sugar from body stores. The liver is the manufacturer of sugar; with fasting or exercise it steps up its output. Studies of prolonged fasting show that body metabolism decreases and more energy is drawn from fat deposits in order to conserve valuable protein and water. Thus, the body functions adaptively under food deprivation in an attempt to get the most out of its available energy sources.

The bulimarexic, in her chronic binge/purge ritual, often creates such an "energy crisis." Physicians with whom we have collaborated consistently express concern over the serious depletion of the bulimarexic's energy reserves. As a result of this depletion, the metabolic rate may decrease to the point where a patient is chronically lethargic. Such a state of mind will in time foster pessimism and inactivity, common precursors to a major problem among bulimarexics: depression.

Psychotropic Drugs

Bulimarexics who seek help are occasionally given drugs that are classified as psychotropic; that is, they affect psychic functioning and/or experience. Among them are phenothiazine derivatives

(Compazine, Phenergan, Stelazine, Temeral, Thorazine), the tricyclic antidepressants (Elavil, Tofranil, and Triavil), and the newer selective seretonin reuptake inhibitors (SSRI's) Prozac, Zoloft, Paxil, to mention a few of the better known drugs. These newer drugs as well as the old standbys such as Elavil are about equally effective in treating many types of depression. However, their efficacy in treating eating disorders is questionable. Some of these drugs are known to increase carbohydrate food craving and enhance bingeing, while others have weight gain as a side effect. Patients who are taking them may mimic the kind of binge eating associated with bulimarexia. Both anorexics and bulimarexics are frightened by an increase in appetite and unexpected weight gain. It reinforces their worst fear: that they will lose control and become "fat." It may also encourage desperate purging practices and noncompliance in taking medication.

Certain medications are dangerous to administer to this population and can even result in death. In the mid 1980s a twenty-three-year-old nursing student, a chronic vomiter, was given lithium while participating in a sleep research study conducted by the National Institutes of Health. During screening, this young woman failed to reveal that she engaged in binge vomiting, which resulted in two distinct bouts of cardiac arrest and an ensuing two-day coma. In general, lithium can predispose toward cardiac arrhythmias, a problem compounded by a loss of potassium from the body. This side effect presents no problem for those who eat regularly and do not resort to vomiting. However, in the case of this chronic vomiter, the loss of stomach acid apparently led to a compensatory loss of extracellular potassium, which doctors believe resulted in cardiac arrest and her death. Lithium should be administered to bulimarexics only under close medical supervision—if at all. Such findings are particularly relevant to the binger and her therapist and serve to underline the tremendous risk of drug treatment. Lithium is particularly risky with anorexics because of the possibility of rapid toxicity from severely restricted fluid intake.

In inpatient settings minor tranquilizers are often prescribed for reducing the tension surrounding eating. However, the benzodiazapines (such as Valium) have a high potential for dependency in these vulnerable clients who have a propensity for addictive behaviors.

In our experience, drugs are rarely effective in attenuating or eliminating bulimarexic or anorexic behavior. During 1985, eighty-four of our clients had been taking Tofranil, Elavil, or Nardil for over a year. Only three reported that drugs had a positive effect on the frequency, intensity, or duration of bingeing or purging. A widely reported 1985 study on imipramine (Tofranil) yielded results that did at first seem promising—so much so that the drug was prominently mentioned in *New Hope for Binge Eaters* by James Hudson and Harrison Pope of Harvard. However, in a two-year follow-up study apparently only three patients remained free of the behavior.

Tofranil, like all tricyclic antidepressants, can cause irregular heartbeat in susceptible individuals. Dr. Randy Sansone, an expert on the physiological consequences of eating disorders, advocates monitoring patients carefully while they are on antidepressant therapy since the presence of an electrolyte disturbance in combination with Tofranil can be precarious.

In the 1990s two developments were of particular significance for eating-disordered women. On the one hand, clinicians seemed more pessimistic about drugs demonstrating efficacy. On the other hand, the SSRIs burst upon the scene with much hype and the promise of being the true "magic bullet" for eating disorders.

In their book *Anorexia Nervosa: A Multidimensional Perspective* (1982), Paul Garfinkel and David Garner concluded: "Many drug therapies have been tried either as the major focus of treatment or as adjuncts to general support and psychological therapies. While some medications may prove beneficial to individual patients, it must be stated that their value is rather limited." In 1985 Arnold Anderson, M.D., of the Johns Hopkins Medical School, reviewed the need for medications and concluded that medications prescribed for weight gain in the anorexic were misguided and their use should be carefully studied. The practice at Johns Hopkins is to wait until weight is restored and then to treat depressive symptoms if they persist.

Peggy Claude-Pierre, who runs the Montreux Counselling Centre for anorexics in British Columbia, is even more critical. When clients arrive at her clinic, they are usually taking four or five psychoactive medications: "They start out being prescribed one; then the doctor adds a second to compensate for the side effects of the first, and a third to compensate for those of the second, and so on." She goes on to say that in well over 90 percent of the cases, the symptoms for which the medication was initially prescribed disappear as clients experience weight restoration, nutritional rehabilitation, and a reversal of their thinking via cognitive therapy.

The American Psychiatric Association in *Practice Guidelines for Eating Disorders* concluded:

(1) Malnourished depressed patients are more prone to side effects and less responsive to antidepressant medications than other patients with depression; (2) Tricyclic antidepressants may add to the risk of hypotension and arrhythmia in anorexia nervosa patients, particularly in purging anorexia nervosa patients, whose hydration may be inadequate and whose cardiac status may be nutritionally compromised; and (3) Some symptoms of depression remit with weight gain.

When Prozac (Fluoxetine) emerged, it was said to have powerful anorectic agents in obese clients, and Eli Lilly tried unsuccessfully to have the drug approved for the treatment of obesity. In the meantime, a spate of articles and impressive double-blind studies appeared. In an eight-week, multicenter, placebo-controlled, randomized trial comparing Fluoxetine 20mg/day, Fluoxetine 60mg/day, and placebo in 387 women with bulimia, the Fluoxetine Bulimia Nervosa Study Group found that overall, Fluoxetine *60mg/daily* was superior to placebo in resisting both binge eating and vomiting (*ArchGen Psychiatry,* 1992; 49[2:139.147]). As a result of these studies, Prozac was cleared for marketing by the Food and Drug Administration in November 1996 for the treatment of bulimia nervosa.

Since the mid-1990s numerous bulimarexic clients who were taking 60mg of Prozac have sought therapy for bingeing and purging. In our experience, a significant number have had great diffi-culty tolerating this higher dosage. Unfortunately many continue their binge/purge cycle, with the medication often contributing to some relief of depressive symptoms but no attenuation of the eat-ing disorder. In addition, we (and many of our colleagues) began to observe a disconcerting, totally unexpected, and devastating side effect: Recovered bulimarexics began to experience significant weight gain! Initially they had a slight weight loss (five or so pounds) which peaked around sixteen to twenty weeks; but after approximately six months, weight gain as high as fifteen to twenty pounds was not uncommon in spite of conscientious eating habits, an absence of bingeing and purging, and consistent exercise. These very vulnerable clients were returning to therapy, desperate for help. A few tried to stop taking Prozac and lost weight but had a return of depressive symptomology. It became another unfortunate catch-22 situation.

A (January 1998) cover story in *Primary Psychiatry* by N. Suss-man, M.D. and David Ginsberg, M.D. addressed these surprising findings and wondered whether the beneficial effects of SSRIs on appetite and weight had been overstated just as the side effects of sleep disturbance and sexual dysfunction may have been underre-ported and underestimated. They concluded that "there is a grow-ing clinical impression . . . suggesting weight gain should be added to the list of SSRI side effects." Once again hopes of a new magic bullet drug for the treatment of eating disorders have not held up.

There are also political issues to consider here when prescribing drugs becomes the answer to women's problems. Over 73 percent of prescriptions for psychotropic drugs are issued to women. Car-olyn Morell, a group counselor who works with women dependent on prescription drugs, points out: "Drugs reinforce women's help-lessness by privatizing and depoliticizing problems and misdefin-ing them as 'metabolic' or 'psychogenic.' . . . In this context, significant drug dependency among women is not surprising."

Many of our clients have admitted taking higher doses of drugs than were prescribed. A few have overdosed and almost died. We are alarmed when such medication is used to treat a psychosocial disorder in women who have already demonstrated their vulnerability to addictive behaviors.

Psychological Factors

There are other adverse consequences of bingeing, primary among them anxiety and depression (created by astronomical food bills, lying, stealing, and isolation) as well as severe stomach pains, headaches, and dizziness. These bodily sensations, painful in their own right, often lead to serious accidents. For example, after gorging on junk food one evening, one woman experienced violent abdominal cramping and a severe headache; in a frantic attempt to return to her apartment, she fell in front of a car. She was taken to the hospital with multiple fractures and a life-threatening concussion!

Severe self-criticism, resentment, and other forms of punishment are also characteristic after bingeing. The ensuing depressive episodes often motivate the woman to seek help. When we reexamined the records of 150 of our clients, we discovered that over 40 percent of them had earlier sought therapy for depression. Of all the consequences of bingeing, depression may prove to be the most frequent and debilitating. We see more and more desperate women who have made suicide gestures and attempts associated with the binge/purge ritual.

THE PURGE

Purging, by whatever means, becomes ritualized and tenacious. Bulimarexics report that purgative methods become relatively effortless as time goes on so that the purges increase in frequency, intensity, and duration. Purging appears to be more deleterious physiologically than bingeing, although bingeing inevitably sets the stage for purging and assumes the central role. There are those who assert that if bingeing can be eliminated, purging will no longer occur. This is simply not the case. In fact, several of our clients reported that they rarely overate (by anyone's standards), yet they purged routinely after consuming modest amounts of food. The purge had been adopted as the most "effective" way to prevent weight gain.

Most bulimarexic women have at one time or another stopped purging, yet they continue to overeat or binge uncontrollably. If the bulimarexic is to free herself from her disorder completely and permanently, she must be prepared to relinquish *both* habits and learn to fortify herself with new, more adaptive habits that satisfy the same needs that maintained her cyclical ritual.

Self-induced Vomiting

Among three hundred bulimarexics we recently interviewed, the frequency of purging by self-induced vomiting varied from once weekly to eighteen times per day. Those who had vomited daily for five or more years often said that they suffered from reverse peristalsis (involuntary intestinal contractions), a condition involving spontaneous regurgitation of the stomach contents. This uncontrollable, painful behavior serves to stimulate more frequent purging so that many felt they had trouble keeping any food down for more than a few minutes.

According to a study by Jill Carni, a Boston psychotherapist who specializes in eating disorders, published in the *Journal of the Massachusetts Dental Society,* chronic vomiting can erode dental enamel, particularly on the inner surface of the teeth, because of the hydrochloric acid content of vomit. Erosion is usually noted on back biting/grinding surfaces and front teeth and increases both the sensitivity of the teeth to changes in temperature and the erosion of the surface of the teeth so that fillings actually protrude and spaces develop between teeth. All of these changes are irreversible, so the bulimarexic's personal appearance, her raison d'etre, may be affected. This erosion can be compounded by a diet limited to citrus fruits and may also result in severe gum disease, innumerable cavities, and tooth loss—which is also augmented by the heightened sugar intake and poor nutritional habits so common among anorexics.

Vomiting has also led to severe tearing and bleeding in and around the esophagus. Hiatal hernias (when the stomach pushes through the diaphragm, creating the sensation of heartburn) and severely infected salivary glands are also commonly reported. One dental hygienist indicated that twenty of her patients, *all* of whom were women, had been eventually forced to undergo salivary, or parotid gland, surgery. Thus, the dentist, not the physician or psychotherapist, may be the first to encounter the ramifications of bulimarexic behavior.

More serious consequences of forced vomiting may also occur. Constant irritation from hydrochloric acid may eventually cause the development of Barrett's esophagus, which involves a change in the epithelial lining of the esophagus, a change that has the potential to advance to cancer. In a recent Swedish study of heartburn related to acid reflux, patients were eight times more likely to develop cancer of the esophagus.

Women who pass out because of purging and who are brought to the hospital for resuscitation face further risks, such as congestive heart failure resulting from overzealous fluid replacement, especially if the attending physicians are unaware (as is usually the case) that the woman is bulimarexic and deficient in potassium.

Hypokalemia

The poor nutrition and restricted salt and mineral intake that often accompany chronic vomiting may result in a deficiency state referred to as *hypokalemia* (potassium deficiency). Potassium is necessary for adequate muscle functioning, and a deficiency is often marked by muscle fatigue, weakness, numbness, erratic heartbeat, kidney damage, and, in severe instances, paralysis. Low levels of potassium can be brought about by chronic vomiting or diuretic abuse. The loss of potassium-containing foods and stomach acids by vomiting serves to precipitate additional imbalances that, in extreme cases, involve sodium and severe dehydration. This deficiency of sodium and potassium in turn creates an electrolyte imbalance. These deficiency states can require immediate medical intervention. A nationally known athlete recently referred to us by her internist had fainted during an important competition after chronic self-induced vomiting had drastically lowered her potassium level. Despite this life-threatening experience, she had withheld critical information from her physician. It was not until she entered our group that she admitted the severity and duration of her purging behavior. Early signs of hypokalemia should be taken seriously since severe hypokalemia may result in cardiac arrhythmia and death!

Kidney problems are another probable consequence of an electrolyte imbalance. In 1979 *Psychological Medicine* published an article by Dr. Gerald Russell of the Department of Psychiatry, Royal Free Hospital, London, describing a patient suffering from what Russell refers to as "bulimia nervosa" (his term for bulimarexia), who developed kidney failure and hypertension after eight years of self-induced vomiting. A kidney transplant was ultimately required, and upon recovery the patient still resorted to occasional bouts of vomiting. Epilepticlike seizure patterns as well as extreme muscle tetany (spasm) were also noted among some of his patients with extreme electrolyte imbalances. Serum potassium levels are crucial, and metabolic monitoring and potassium supplementation may be necessary to prevent kidney failure.

Laxative and Diuretic Abuse

The most hazardous methods of weight control include laxative and diuretic abuse. As Dr. Randy Sansone aptly points out in his recent overview of destructive weight-loss methods, many complications can be detected during a routine physical examination. In the first edition of this book, we reported that purging with laxatives or diuretics seemed to be on the increase. In 1978 the majority of bulimarexics (83 percent) we surveyed were vomiters. However, just two years later, by 1980, less than 68 percent relied on self-induced vomiting; laxative and diuretic purges were considered easier to conceal and generally less painful than chronic vomiting.

Fortunately, since that time, our surveys suggest that, with the help of responsible journalism, the dangers of extreme laxative abuse are now receiving attention. Bulimarexics are beginning to realize that laxatives are not only ineffective in controlling weight but potentially toxic. Stimulant laxatives such as Ex-Lax, Evac-U-Gen, and Correctol may cause abdominal cramping, nausea, vomiting, and bloating. With chronic laxative abuse, the lower colon, especially the ascending colon and the terminal ileum, may undergo pathologic changes. There may be a loss of normal mucosa, dilation and distention of the colon accompanied by atrophy and thinning of mucosal and muscular layers, along with the development of multiple ulcers. Medically, the condition is called cathartic colon. In its extreme form, a colectomy (removal of the colon) may be necessary. Another condition directly caused by chronic laxative abuse, melanosis coli, in which the mucosa of the lower bowel and rectum is turned black by chronic use of laxatives, has also been reported.

Furthermore, recurring localized or generalized skin rashes can result from overuse of the phenolphthalein-type laxatives such as Ex-Lax, Correctol, and Feenamint. Inflammation followed by a brownish-gray discoloration of the skin that tends to darken with each dose is characteristic of this condition. A physician should, of course, be consulted.

Laxatives such as castor oil serve to liquify feces and act as irritants that increase peristalsis. In doing so, they reduce the ability of the intestines to absorb fluids and may actually prevent intestinal action. Epsom salts, on the other hand, tends to increase volume within the intestines by attracting fluid so that the gut swells. As a result, food is more rapidly eliminated. Mineral oils lubricate and thereby prevent fecal water from being reabsorbed as it passes through intestines. This in turn prevents the body from absorbing vitamins such as E, A, D, and K.

Diuretics (water pills) rid the body of water and if taken in amounts that exceed recommended dosage can cause serious dehydration. During the premenstrual period when the level of estrogen rises, women generally gain weight due to water retention, characterized by puffiness, particularly around the face and feet. Diuretics are often used to stimulate urination in order to relieve this swelling; and overuse leads to dehydration. In response, the kidneys reduce the amount of water and salt excreted from the body. Again, dehydration resulting from restricted food intake and chronic diuretic abuse often leads to a deficiency of sodium and potassium that in turn creates an electrolyte imbalance. The kidneys then retain sodium at the expense of potassium, which is slowly excreted. The final result is muscle weakness, numbness, and, ultimately, paralysis. Physicians may prescribe diuretics for women who have severe premenstrual difficulties, but bulimarexics are likely to exaggerate symptoms in order to receive medication. Physicians need to be aware of this.

Dehydration and electrolyte imbalances due to increased potassium loss through the gastrointestinal tract can also result from prolonged laxative abuse. Chronic abusers typically suffer severe constipation because of the loss of intestinal muscle tone and increasing dependency upon laxatives. An alarming number of women have acknowledged consumption of over *fifty laxatives daily* in an attempt to maintain bowel control. Abuse of irritant laxatives—such as castor oil and cascara—over a period of years can also produce severe intestinal abnormalities that simulate inflammatory bowel disease.

Here a vicious cycle has been set up. Because the intestine has been thoroughly emptied, a bowel movement may not take place for days. Bulimarexics, assuming that they are constipated, resort to more laxatives. Since prolonged irritation and stimulation can cause intestinal muscles to become dependent upon laxatives for contraction, the laxative abuser will often feel bloated or experience gas or stomach pain. X-rays may reveal a transient narrowing of the intestine similar to that of patients suffering from ulcerative colitis. In some cases, but by no means all, these abnormalities may be partially reversed when the irritant laxatives are discontinued.

How can such serious problems develop? Quite simply, when purging becomes habitual—regardless of how it is accomplished— the purger, typically dehydrated and hungry, eats and drinks more.

Feeling full, she then reinitiates the cycle and purges once again. Along the way the binge becomes associated with numerous environmental cues that reinforce the urge to binge or purge.

Ipecac Ingestion

Syrup of ipecac, useful as an antidote to poison or drug overdose, produces vomiting, usually within a half hour. Ipecac works by stimulating the vomiting center in the brainstem and by irritating the gastrointestinal tract. Because it induces vomiting and is readily available over-the-counter, it has become a common purgative. When taken in excess (15 to 20 cc) or if vomiting fails to occur, the person can experience chest pain, rapid heart rate, shortness of breath, and electrocardiogram abnormalities that can persist for weeks even after discontinuation of the substance. Chronic abuse may lead to bloody diarrhea, stomach pain, convulsions, heart failure, and eventually shock and death. Fortunately, recent media attention has done much to reduce the abuse of syrup of ipecac.

Secondary Amenorrhea

Secondary amenorrhea, or cessation of menstruation, is not unusual among bulimarexics. Undernourishment is a likely factor here. Dr. Rose Frisch, in her research on fatness and reproduction, has shown that established menstrual function is disturbed when fat levels drop below about 22 percent of body weight. Weight fluctuation in this critical range and undernourishment from purging may well account for the menstrual irregularity so often reported by bulimarexics, particularly those who purge by fasting and/or extreme dieting. The menstrual cycle can also be interrupted by environmental stress, a primary factor in bulimarexia. Regardless of the underlying cause, however, a causal relationship exists among body weight, stress, and the onset or regularity of menstruation. As Dr. Vincent points out, "Among dancers who binge and purge, 'thinness'—in and of itself or along with the

'stresses' of dancing—may be responsible for the lack of maintenance of a regular menstrual cycle."

Dr. Christopher Cann and his colleagues at the University of
California, San Francisco, reported that young women who suffer
from amenorrhea may have less bone density than normal and are
at greater risk of stress fractures. (This condition, called *osteoporosis*, represents a major health threat to older women.) The young
women in Dr. Cann's study all suffered from hypothalamic amenorrhea, in which the hormone that causes menstruation is not produced; after four or five years of amenorrhea, significant bone loss
can occur. Several new drugs, such as Fosamax, show promise in replacing this critical loss. Exercise and strength training *may* deter
bone loss but cannot prevent this extremely serious condition. Bulimarexics and others who are amenorrheic should consult with a
gynecologist for the best individual treatment.

Because bulimarexics have often avoided physicians and their
symptoms have gone unrecognized, there is little longitudinal research with regard to menstrual irregularities. What are the long-
term effects on the reproductive system? Are fertility and
childbearing affected? Does menstruation return spontaneously
with proper nutrition and other therapy? We have no definitive answers to these questions. We do know that many bulimarexics begin
to menstruate normally once they abandon their bizarre behavior
and develop other means of stress reduction. So there is cause for
optimism if women will begin to talk freely with their physicians.

The following letter from one of our clients illustrates many of
the problems and potential ramifications of bingeing and purging.
This woman agreed to let us use her history, as told in her own
words:

Dear Drs. White:

For the first five of my seven years as a bulimarexic, I experienced occasional dizzy spells, headaches, stomach cramps, and the obvious negative reactions from laxative abuse. However, the summer of my fifth year
marked the beginning of serious problems that would increase until I
finally gave up this abusive habit.

I had been terribly depressed. I was in what I considered to be a "fat" period. Liquid protein diets were the "in" thing that summer and I felt this was my answer. I began ingesting supplements of this vile substance, but continued to use a diuretic as I felt this all-liquid diet would make me bloated. Needless to say, I was playing [Russian] roulette! It was only a matter of time before I was so weak and lethargic I could barely function, even on a schedule of light activity. I became more depressed even though the sight of weight coming off usually boosted my spirits enough to keep up my abusive ritual.

One day I was driving to visit my sister. I became so dizzy that my vision was blurred, and I began shaking. I actually feared for my life! I somehow managed to get to my sister's house, although the last thing I should have been doing was operating a car. I remember telling my sister I really needed a glass of orange juice. She asked me if I was sick [and said] I looked terrible! All I could see was that I looked thin!! Anyway, I stayed at her house until I began feeling better and felt able to return home. As soon as I got home, however, I felt so faint that I was scared to be alone. I drove myself to the emergency room of the hospital. I told them I was having dizzy spells, felt faint, and just wanted to be sure I didn't have "some sort of virus." I was so good at concealing the cause of my suffering.

The doctor on duty took my blood pressure, some blood samples, and made the routine checks that I guess all emergency patients receive. After a few minutes the lab reports were back. The doctor looked at me and said, "No wonder you feel so lousy, you're barely alive." I knew he wasn't kidding. He then began to tell me that I had a potassium deficiency. I was anemic and lacking in all sorts of important minerals. I was so afraid of being "discovered" that I took the news as if I had caught something dreadful from the air! He then began to ask me about my medical history—what had I possibly done to cause this reaction? I was a master at avoiding any answer which would implicate me as a laxative abuser. Finally, he asked the key question: "Have you been dieting strenuously?" I was sure he knew enough from my lab reports to figure this one out. I decided to be partially honest. "Well, yes," I answered, "I have been dieting very seriously." He then threw up his hands and in disgust said, "You damn women and your diets; don't you know that your body must have a minimum of nutrients to survive?" I said yes, and that I should have been taking a vitamin supplement. He laughed and said that I'd have to take a lot more than a vitamin pill to regain normal status and proceeded to write me prescriptions for potassium and [other] supplements, megavitamins, iron, and folic acid.

I left feeling relieved that I was still well enough to go home and not be hospitalized, but really shaken by the entire experience. I look back on this now and remember how relieved I was that he hadn't discovered that I was severely bulimarexic at that time. I was very careful after that. I took my medicine faithfully, went back for my check-up lab tests, and breathed a sigh of relief. I did not, however, stop bingeing and purging at that point. I just began to eat again, threw out the liquid protein, and purged less often for a while.

Two years later, I began having difficulty when I urinated. Thinking I had a bladder infection or cystitis, I went to my doctor to have it checked out. When he looked at me, he said he didn't think I had a bladder infection but that I seemed to have a great deal of acidity in my urine, which caused the burning sensation I had been experiencing. He was also concerned that it might have something to do with a low-grade infection, which could have caused the urinary problem.

I left his office in complete disgust. I had done this! I knew it was from abusing diuretics and laxatives. This was my breaking point. I had gone down as far as I could go. I was so depressed and disgusted with the entire habit that I was determined to turn my life and what health I had left around. I knew I had to get treatment.

I stopped bingeing in September, right after our workshop. Every year I remember the date as one remembers something wonderful, an anniversary. However, I had no way of knowing that my seven years of abuse would continue to plague me for some time.

Fifteen months after I had completely stopped bingeing and purging, I had major abdominal surgery for a tumor. My immediate fear was that I had caused this with laxatives. I decided to tell all—to share my entire bulimarexic history with my physician. He was a wonderful listener. Patiently, he sat as I went through my story. By the end I was crying. I remember telling him that for fifteen months I had been so "good" and that I had to know if I had done this to myself. He told me that it was something that could never really be answered, but that the body has strange ways of scarring and healing itself after trauma. He said that although he wasn't sure if bulimarexia actually caused the tumor, he felt that through years of abuse of this area, I might have weakened it enough to make it more susceptible to injury or disease. He tried hard to reassure me that I had not necessarily done this to myself, but I am not convinced.

After my lengthy recovery from colon surgery, I began to learn more about the entire elimination system of the body. I found that there were many possible side effects from laxative abuse even after the laxatives had been stopped. In many ways, I consider myself a "guinea pig" to the physical recovery of laxative abuse. When the colon has become laxative dependent, it ceases to function in the same way a normal colon would. The muscles within the walls of the colon can atrophy, and the large sphincter muscle at the base of the anus loses normal control and does not expand and contract normally. This often leads to the embarrassment of loss of bowel control, which is common among long-term laxative abusers.

In addition, the colon is set up to remove fecal matter in a consistent motion or rhythm. When laxatives are taken, the natural rhythm is upset, and . . . the colon's synchronization becomes irregular. This often causes painful spasms. In order for the colon to eliminate waste products, there must be specific bacteria to enable the gases that build up to move the waste material along and cause the proper chain reaction. When laxatives are used, a lot of this necessary bacteria is washed out. It takes approximately three days for this bacteria to build back up to the level necessary for proper elimination. Because laxatives pull water from the system, the laxative abuser is often in danger of becoming dehydrated. Therefore, in an attempt to maintain normal fluid levels, the body will begin to store water; thus the laxative abuser often complains about feeling bloated. In extreme cases this can lead to cathartic colon, which is a condition that is caused by chronic use of laxatives. It impairs absorption of water and causes bloating, distention, and pain in the lower abdomen.

When a bulimarexic or laxative abuser decides to give up this damaging habit, there are important physical considerations. When I stopped taking laxatives, I stopped "cold turkey." After seven years of abuse, I quite simply stopped taking them at all. This abrupt change was not in the best interest of my recovery, which I found out the hard way. To break the laxative habit requires great determination and patience. For the first several weeks, bloating and a heavy sensation is a common complaint. So, many women go back to laxatives "just one more time." They are back to square one. It is very important for the recovering bulimarexic to realize that it may take up to ten days before the natural action of the colon is reestablished. Breaking the habit is definitely worth the wait!

Diet is another aspect of recovery. When I stopped taking laxatives, I began to eat a high-fiber diet. I found myself in great distress, and had a lot of trouble with cramps and bloating. I later discovered that the colon must be reintroduced to fiber very gradually and that a low-fiber diet is recommended for the first few weeks until the symptoms begin to dissipate. The fiber intake for a normal diet is recommended to be 25 to 30g of fiber a day. Although one of the most uncomfortable symptoms will be the bloating and waterlogged feeling, it is essential to drink a minimum of six and better still eight glasses of water a day to help the body eliminate the excess fluid. Drinking water actually aids the process, even though it seems a contradiction in terms!

I have shared my healing process with many laxative abusers and found it to be the safest and most reliable method. I do not recommend stopping laxatives abruptly but rather slowly decreasing the number while following a low-fiber diet and drinking plenty of water over a period of several weeks. After laxative use has completely stopped, continue on the low-fiber regime for another full week, and then begin slowly adding fiber to the diet. It may take months for full regularity to resume, depending on how laxatives have been used and in what amount. The colon can and will heal itself and work normally again if given time and patience along with healthy food and plenty of liquids. I would also recommend consulting a good gastroenterologist if after several weeks of proper eating normal bowel function has not been restored.

A number of dietary considerations will help the recovering laxative abuser and here are some of them.

Beverages: Drink decaffeinated coffee, weak or herb tea, carbonated beverages, fruit juice. Restrict milk products because they add to the problem of bloating and gas.
Meat, Fish, Poultry: Any lean cut is all right. Avoid seasoned or highly spiced meats.
Eggs: Best if not combined with milk.
Cheese: Hard cheeses are best. Cottage cheese and many softer cheeses often produce gas.
Breads: White, light whole wheat, rye (seedless), crackers, melba toast. Avoid whole-grain breads, especially with seeds.
Cereals: Oatmeal, Cream of Wheat, Wheatena, dry cereals without bran, rice noodles, spaghetti, macaroni. Avoid bran, whole grains, granola, added nuts, brown rice.
Vegetables: All vegetables should be cooked or lightly steamed. Do not eat

vegetables raw or with skins or seeds. Vegetables best avoided because of the gas they produce are: cabbage, cauliflower, onions, radishes, broccoli, brussels sprouts, green peppers. Excellent foods to eat to help eliminate fluid buildup are: asparagus, mushrooms, and parsley.
Fruit: No raw fruits, skins, or seeds. Bananas are fine, or any cooked fruit such as applesauce, canned pears, peaches.
Extras: Spices and seasonings in moderation, chocolate, mayonnaise, smooth peanut butter, plain cookies, cake, gelatin, pastries without a lot of added milk.

The idea is to slowly reintroduce the colon to bulk foods while lessening the gas pains. Then fiber can gradually be introduced to the diet. The eventual goal is to reach maximum health and normal elimination through proper diet, not artificial stimulants. It is important to drink six to eight glasses of water every day.

ANOREXIA NERVOSA: MEDICAL IMPLICATIONS

Endocrine Complications

The entire endocrine system is compromised by starvation. Some 80 percent of clients with eating disorders develop a cessation of menses when their total body fat is reduced to less than 20 percent of their total body weight. As a consequence, amenorrhea is considered to be one of the primary features of anorexia nervosa and is associated with hypothalamic dysfunction. Women and girls with anorexia nervosa have significantly lower levels of both female and male hormones (Van-Binsberger, et al., 1990).

A resumption of menses occurs in anorexics when their weight reaches approximately 90 percent of their standard body weight. The hypothalamic—pituitary—ovarian function returns to normal with resumption of menses. Serum estradiol (an estrogen hormone) levels rise as menses returns. Puberty, including the onset of periods, may be delayed in adolescents with anorexia nervosa, leading to stopped or delayed growth.

Significant osteoporosis is present in over 50 percent of women with anorexia nervosa, and estrogen administration or hormone replacement alone does not prevent bone loss. The adult anorexia nervosa individual has marked *spinal osteopenia* (abnormally low bone density) when bone loss is compared to age-matched normal women. Women with an onset of amenorrhea before age eighteen had significantly lower spinal bone density than women who developed amenorrhea later.

There have been conflicting studies about whether osteopenia improves or persists after clients overcome anorexia nervosa. The duration of amenorrhea was the best predictor of reduced bone density, and women with a longer duration of amenorrhea showed less recovery of their osteoporosis (Ward et al. 1997).

According to Joan Ryan (1995), elite athletes are forced to race against puberty to maintain the "ideal shape and size." Round, tall gymnasts or ice skaters do not win. Those who starve themselves have been found to have bone densities of postmenopausal women in their sixties and seventies and as a result are much more susceptible to stress fractures. The combination of low bone density and riskier and more demanding routines, such as the now-expected triple jumps in ice skating, are crippling and killing more and more young women athletes.

Thyroid function tests in the anorexic often appear grossly abnormal. All circulating levels of thyroxine (T4) and triodothyronine (T3) are low and are the hallmark of starvation—reducing the metabolic rate to conserve calories.

Renal Complications

Anorexics suffer abnormalities in water balance because they restrict fluids. This leads to the serious complications of dehydration, especially in hot weather. As previously noted, chronic potassium depletion can lead to hypokalemia and kidney failure and/or cardiac arrhythmia and death.

When anorexics try to "make weight," they can overload themselves with fluids, a condition called *hyponatrenia* that can be serious enough to cause cerebral edema (water on the brain) and seizures.

Gastrointestinal Complications

Anorexics frequently complain about bloating and abdominal pain, which can be major obstacles as they become willing to eat more and gain weight. They also frequently suffer from delayed gastric emptying, unbearable feelings of fullness, belching, gas, and constipation. These problems underline the importance of medical monitoring by a physician who can prescribe drugs to ease these side effects.

A serious life-threatening complication of refeeding can be the spontaneous rupture of the stomach. In a review of sixty-six cases by Saul et al. (1981), eleven were anorexics undergoing refeeding. Another painful condition called *refeeding pancreatitis* can also occur.

Cardiopulmonary Complications

Electrocardiograms of anorexic clients are frequently abnormal. Bradycardia (slow heartbeat) and hypotension (abnormally low blood pressure) are common, reflecting the body's adaptive metabolic response to starvation. Impairment of ventricular function, arrhythmias, and a decrease in cardiac chamber dimensions are some of the serious life-threatening complications. Muscle tissue in the heart lacks oxygen and in response reduces its output leading to a slow heart rate and EKG changes. Often there is a thinning of the heart muscle wall as well. Extremities are always cold because of diminished blood circulation. The body tries to shut down or slow down to save itself. Cardiac functioning can return to normal with nutritional rehabilitation, but rapid refeeding and/or excessive exercise can be extremely dangerous for an already seriously compromised cardiovascular system. Sudden cardiac arrest and death can occur, as in the tragic case of singer Karen Carpenter, who battled bulimia and anorexia for years.

Eating Disorders and Nutritional Implications

In our early group treatment of bulimarexics, we did not encourage women to use their therapy time to discuss food because the sessions invariably shifted to contests as to who was the "biggest and baddest binger." Many of our student clients then were nutrition majors who were obviously aware of the basics of good nutrition but failed to adhere to them. Once the process of recovery was under way, we did introduce nutritional counseling through an outside resource. At that point the women seemed much more receptive to learning how to eat normally.

Later we began to read accounts of studies about the impact of starvation and dieting on human and animal subjects. The research suggested that repeated dieting could result in altered metabolism, making it more and more difficult to lose weight. We began to wonder if many of the behaviors we saw in bulimarexic women could be the result of undernutrition and/or malnutrition rather than the cause. Albert Stunkard, a University of Pennsylvania obesity expert, and his colleagues raised similar questions about obesity and asked whether the emotional disorders so closely linked to obesity were the result of dieting rather than the cause of obesity. Today's obesity research has taken, in Stunkard's words, a "180-degree change of direction" as these speculations have been confirmed. Our thinking about bulimarexia has also undergone significant modification.

The most systematic and extensive study related to starvation ever undertaken was carried out during the mid-1940s with thirty-six men at the University of Minnesota. Conscientious objectors, they agreed to participate in the nine-month study as an alternative to military service. For the first three months of the experiment, the men were fed normal amounts of food while their behavior, personalities, and eating patterns were studied closely. For the next three months they were restricted to about half of their former food intake and lost about 26 percent of their original body weight. The total number of calories during the semistarvation phase was 1,660 per day, provided in three nutritious meals with vitamin supplements. The men were then refed a full intake for three months and observed for a period beyond the conclusion of the experiment.

Dramatic physical, psychological, and social changes occurred. What is most striking is that these changes were observed not only during the starvation phase but also during the rehabilitation phase. In the starvation phase, the men were obsessed with food. Many began reading cookbooks and exchanging recipes. Nearly 40 percent wanted to improve their cooking skills when the study was over, and a few even changed their occupations to chef. They spent most of their days planning how to eat their allotment of food, with a demand for hot, spicy foods, and began to drink so much coffee and tea that they had to be limited to nine cups per day. Several men engaged in binge eating followed by vomiting. The majority reported constant hunger.

There were also significant emotional changes. The men became irritable and apathetic. The fastidious among them neglected personal hygiene. Emotional distress increased. Two subjects slipped into psychotic disturbances. Fighting, weeping, thoughts of suicide, and violence were also noted. The men lost their sense of humor, and social contacts declined. They began to isolate themselves, lost sexual interest, and became tired, weak, and listless. Dizziness, headaches, reduced strength, and poor motor control were frequent symptoms. They were always cold and hypersensitive to light.

At the end of the semistarvation phase, the men were rehabilitated over a period of twelve weeks. What transpired during this period was even more intriguing. They often found themselves out of control when confronted with food: "In many cases the men were not content to eat 'normal menus' but persevered in their habits of making fantastic concoctions and combinations. A free choice of ingredients, moreover, stimulated 'creative' and 'experimental' playing with food . . . licking of plates and neglect of table manners persisted." Many men ate nearly continuously. Even after twelve weeks of refeeding, they seemed insatiable, experiencing an increase in hunger immediately after a large meal. Their gluttony often involved consumption of between eight and ten thousand calories at a time! Some would vomit after such episodes. After about five months of rehabilitation, the majority of the men experienced some normalization of their eating patterns; however, more than eight months later, a few still had disordered responses to food. A subset of these men developed bulimarexia that persisted many months after they were permitted free access to food.

Professor Ancel Keys was the director of this famous starvation study. The information from the study was to help the secretary of war (to whom Keys was an assistant during the war years) in the rehabilitation of starving postwar populations in war zones.

Unfortunately, it took nearly forty years for researchers to resurrect and then apply many of Keys's findings, which are very much in line with current thinking about eating disorders and starvation. Between 1975 and 1985, research findings began to focus on biochemical rather than psychogenic explanations of obesity. Body weight, it appeared, was not easily altered but vigorously defended, and willpower had little to do with weight loss. It was discovered that there was a "set point" within each of us, a range of natural/stable weight that our bodies return to over and over again. The psychological distress of the Keys subjects seems related to the reduction of stores of body fat below the set point, and their disordered response to food was not corrected until fat stores were replenished—*over a year later!* In other words, refeeding and overfeeding alone did not reduce their distress. Researcher Ethan Allen Simms investigated the set point from an opposite view. He wondered what would happen biochemically when individuals were forced to gain weight. The results of this study at the Vermont State Prison provided ammunition for the set-point theory. For two hundred days Simms overfed groups of prisoner volunteers and restricted their exercise. The men all had to double the amount of food they ate, and the majority struggled valiantly to gain twenty pounds. Having attained their goal weight, it was found that the men could only maintain the weight gain by continued overeating. They became apathetic, lethargic, and often threw up after breakfast. After the experiment was over, the majority lost weight effortlessly, returning to their natural or customary weights.

Both the Keys and Simms studies showed clearly how difficult it was to lose as well as gain weight. However, what happens biochemically to bring one's body back to its original set point and what factors might raise or lower set point remained a mystery.

Further research, at Rockefeller University, discovered a raising and lowering of metabolism in a human subject who was asked to gain and then lose twenty pounds. During the gaining phase, he began to burn calories at a furious rate, particularly directly after meals—a metabolic heat production phase called *thermogenesis*. This phenomenon had been observed in the Simms prisoners, who sweated profusely and complained constantly of being hot. When the Rockefeller subject was in the weight-losing phase, his metabolism slowed after meals, and he conserved energy efficiently. In other words, he adjusted his metabolism to counteract deviations from his ideal weight.

Other studies came up with interesting results about the effects of repeated weight gain and loss (now referred to as *yo-yo dieting*). Kelly Brownwell at the University of Pennsylvania, in collaboration with researchers at Vassar, found that rats became more and more food efficient after each diet and, after their second diet, gained weight at three times the rate they did the first time around.

In 1983 two books strongly suggested that continual dieting may be a critical contributing factor in eating disorders. William Bennett and Joel Gurin in *The Dieter's Dilemma: Eating Less and Eating More* cited overwhelming evidence that diets do not and cannot reduce weight permanently. In fact, they found that a rapid five-pound weight loss typically led to a six-pound weight gain with a higher level of body fat introduced with the extra added pound. Thus, dieting actually leads to an increase in the number of fat cells stored. Janet Polivy and C. Peter Herman in *Breaking the Diet Habit: the Natural Weight Alternative* found further direct risks associated with dieting. Dieting, they discovered, led to binge eating. Dieters who were forced to overeat—or simply believed they had overeaten—went on to overeat even more. Instead of eating when they were hungry, dieters seemed to eat for various irra-tional or emotional reasons—their internal body signals and body chemistry became deranged. This reinforced their greatest fear: "I will gain weight if I eat over six hundred calories a day." Dieters also became depressed, irritable, and easily distracted, with ele-vated free fatty acid levels suggesting that they were in a constant state of stress.

If dieting slows metabolism and encourages the body to retain unwanted fat, what can happen to the biochemistry of the buli-marexic who is in a constant state of malnutrition and starvation? One of our colleagues, Dr. Judith Ravar of Paris, who recently vis-ited us on a Fulbright scholarship, writes that the bulimarexic "who eats nothing during the day and binges in the evening is, therefore, stocking energy just before the energy needs for the day disappear, and is surviving the next day on an energy level which is lower than normal. At the same time she is teaching her body to economize on energy and to stock the maximum of fuel." Thus, what started off as an apparently efficient way to *prevent* weight gain paradoxi-cally can soon *lead* to it.

Serendipity Anorexics

The Keys studies confirmed that weeks or months of starving can cause the symptoms of anorexia nervosa and bulimia to be self-perpetuating. I agree wholeheartedly. These findings explain the many young women I have treated whom I call *serendipity anorex-ics* because they were girls or women of normal weight and seem-ingly well adjusted and happy before an event that caused them to lose weight. In many cases it is an illness such as mononucleosis and what starts off as an illness caused by weight loss soon be-comes a full-blown anorexic merry-go-round that they are unable to get off of without professional intervention.

I firmly believe anorexics are under the influence of powerful biological forces that alter their thinking in profound and extraor-dinarily identical ways. Take any group of anorexics and bring them together. Their dialogue, thinking, rituals, goals, and self-perceptions are remarkably similar, just as the symptoms of chicken pox and measles are. Fifteen years ago I had an experience that made me a believer. I became quite ill and almost died of pneumonia. I dropped from my usual accustomed weight of about 130 pounds to 105 pounds. As I began to recover, I was horrified to discover that my thinking, body image disparagement, and body image distortion was very similar to that of my clients. I too was under the impact of starvation.

As has already been mentioned, laxative abuse has also proven ineffective as a means of ridding the body of calories. One hundred and fifty laxative tablets will only account for a little more than one hundred calories—hardly worth the risk that laxative abuse poses. And despite intensified purging, women begin to add pounds. At this point many turn to therapy in desperation—purging as a means of weight control has backfired. Initially we believed purging to be more harmful than bingeing. Now there is evidence that binge eating may be more harmful than being overweight since overeating summons excess insulin that often leads to pancreatic stress. Thus the bulimarexic is in double jeopardy by subjecting her body to bingeing followed by purging.

In our experience, most women who develop eating disorders were close to their normal or stable weight before embarking on diets that eventually led to bingeing and purging or starvation. The research of Drs. Susan and Wayne Wooley suggests that women who are already slim and who attempt to reduce below their set point appear to be at high risk for eating disorders. This is due to reduced metabolic rate that slows weight loss and increases appetite.

UNLESS the clients with eating disorders can be completely honest about the severity of their binge/purge behavior or inability to stop dieting, they can anticipate little help. Many women have reached out to excellent physicians, psychologists, and nutritionists, but it is not enough for them merely to inform their doctors that they have been "dieting heavily" or relying on laxatives, diuretics, or vomiting. Women report, "My doctor will not take me seriously." Inherent in this veiled plea for help is the hope that the doctor will somehow condone the aberrant behavior—and, in fact, that is often what happens. Take Eunice, for example. At a nationally recognized clinic, she was examined by no less than four specialists. Almost all of the adverse medical findings cited in this chapter were present, yet none of these top-flight specialists uncovered her eight-year history of binge vomiting! Eunice was not dishonest— she "mentioned" vomiting to three of the four doctors, but she did not *emphasize* it. Instead of admitting to vomiting approximately two to three times daily after consuming an average of eight to ten thousand calories, Eunice merely stated that she *sometimes* felt bloated after overeating and would vomit uncontrollably. Surprisingly, many physicians are not yet sophisticated about eating disorders, despite the burgeoning interest resulting from articles in the professional and lay press. They are skeptical—apt to shake their heads in disbelief. The same is often true of the anorexic in her initial stages. Many physicians overlook the loss of a few pounds instead of monitoring it—and of course managed care is creating more pressure to get patients in and out quickly. Psychological problems and the study of nutrition have only recently become a significant part of the medical school curriculum in the United States. Many doctors have learned to probe, yet they are also aware of the importance of establishing rapport in a relatively short period of time. This is not to excuse the physician who matter-of-factly dismisses important diagnostic cues with such statements as, "The way you look, you don't have to worry about your weight!" But doctors are not clairvoyant nor can they be expected to be.

As a result of our group work, we have established a referral system with physicians and nurse-practitioners throughout the country. Some of those involved are practitioners; others are research clinicians; many had eating disorders. All are interested in this pervasive problem and its medical ramifications. At the moment, however, responsibility must rest with the client and those to whom she turns in desperation. We would urge such potential sources of support to *insist* upon regular medical monitoring and insure, whenever possible, that doctors, nutritionists, and therapists are aware of the frequency and duration of binge/purge behavior and self-starvation. On the other hand, professionals who encounter these women must be more assertive, particularly during the initial interview, if treatment is to be effective. The first step must therefore involve early detection in both the anorexic and bulimarexic and referral to appropriate treatment resources.

7.

The Bulimarexic Workshop

TO LAUGH IS TO RISK APPEARING THE FOOL,

TO WEEP IS TO RISK APPEARING SENTIMENTAL,

TO REACH OUT FOR ANOTHER IS TO RISK INVOLVEMENT,

TO EXPOSE FEELINGS IS TO RISK EXPOSING THE SELF,

TO PLACE IDEAS AND DREAMS BEFORE THE CROWD IS TO RISK
    LOSS,

TO LOVE IS TO RISK REJECTION,

TO LIVE IS TO RISK DYING,

TO HOPE IS TO RISK DESPAIR,

TO TRY AT ALL IS TO RISK FAILURE,

BUT RISK WE MUST,

BECAUSE THE GREATEST HAZARD OF ALL IS TO RISK NOTHING,

FOR THOSE WHO RISK NOTHING, DO NOTHING, HAVE NOTHING,

ARE NOTHING.

Group Member

WE have worked with over two thousand women struggling with bulimarexia, and we believe that bulimarexia is a learned behavior. It can therefore be unlearned. By behavior, we mean not only actions but thought processes and attitudes as well. As with many behavioral problems, early detection often facilitates recovery in therapy. Those who came to us when they were just beginning to binge and purge—and were frightened that they might continue—often were able to change their destructive eating habits with relative ease. Some, though not all, could have handled their problems themselves or with a minimum of therapy if they had been familiar with the principles of our treatment program. We hope that this chapter will prove helpful to such women—and to the parents, husbands, lovers, and friends who are wondering what they can do.

Many of the women we see have already had years of individual psychotherapy. Often their therapists have focused on deepseated underlying causes, which did not help the women with the here and now. Some were labeled anorexic and were confronted with clinical descriptions that were foreign and frightening. Others have continued to feel bizarre and alone, even though they were told that their behavior was not uncommon. And there are some who had never admitted to their secret eating behavior. In other words, they did not "own" their bingeing and purging.

The bulimarexics we have met have attempted to deal with their problems in a variety of treatment settings. Individual work with a male or a female therapist is the most usual. Here a combination of behavioral, rational-emotive, gestalt, interpersonal problem-solving, and assertiveness-training techniques seems most beneficial, especially when the therapist understands the way most women are reared in our culture. In one-to-one therapy, female therapists may have better results because women tend to relate to and identify with one another—and also because bulimarexics have an overwhelming tendency to surrender their power to men. In general, these are especially attractive women who are "good patients" in the traditional sense. They want to please, and they rarely challenge a male therapist. As pointed out earlier, few bulimarexic women are completely honest about the frequency, intensity, and duration of the behaviors they yearn to alter.

As we reviewed the progress of these women, we came to feel that individual therapy was not the most effective treatment (in fact, it began to seem the least effective). Our exploratory work soon proved so revealing that we began more intensive group therapy as an alternative to individual work. Initially our groups consisted of twelve to fifteen bulimarexics. We found that this number was too large and began limiting the group to no more than ten women. The group work is intensely demanding, requiring much "after-hours" processing with regard to each participant. The group soon becomes cohesive so that short-term, intensive therapy is ideally suited to addressing specific goals. Since the women come from various areas of the country, there are also logistical and financial considerations, which include travel and leaving families and work responsibilities. In recent years we have adopted a workshop format involving fifteen to twenty hours of therapy over a three-day period. This allows ample time for formal group work, informal risk taking outside of the group, and at the same time reinforces our belief that bulimarexia is a habit rather than a chronic disease process. Special attention is, of course, given to clarifying treatments goals and assuring that those who need follow-up and more extensive professional intervention can receive it.

Who should be treated in this type of group? We feel that the group should be composed of women who are truly bulimarexic. Women suffering from classic anorexia nervosa or obesity are not appropriate to this group experience. Their dynamics are quite different. They cannot identify with the bulimarexic and therefore run the risk of further alienation. Many are in need of medical management and, as such, should not be included.

It might be supposed that successful outcome in treatment is directly related to how long the destructive eating pattern has been going on, to the intensity of gorging and purging, and to the methods these women use to purge. While it is generally true that women in the early stages of bulimarexia recover more quickly, two factors seem far more relevant. The first involves the *level of commitment to change* the woman possesses when she enters treatment. Second, but of equal importance, are the *strategies* she employs to overcome bulimarexia. What can she do in the face of anxiety? What can she substitute for binge eating? If the woman can call upon more productive strategies to cope with the stresses of daily life, she is on her way to recovery. The commitment to initiate and maintain personal growth through alternative behaviors is therefore crucial.

Naming this behavior *bulimarexia* was not something we

wanted to do because such labeling could, in and of itself, be harmful. Labels, unless clearly defined in terms of precise behaviors, often serve as a refuge. They symbolize safe edifices behind which a person can hide and wait to be "cured." In order to avoid this, let us review the primary characteristics of bulimarexia so that women who are suffering from classic anorexia and obesity do not seek treatment that was not intentionally designed for them.

First, the bulimarexic alternately binges on food and then purges, typically by self-induced vomiting, or by abuse of laxatives or diuretics. Although fasting can be another method of purging, it is far less prevalent and should not be confused with the typical anorexic pattern in which the *major emphasis is on starvation.* Second, the bulimarexic is obsessed with not getting fat. For her, actual body weight is far less important than her body proportions and *how she sees herself.* Self-esteem is based primarily upon how she feels she looks so that the successes (or failures) of her life are measured by this yardstick.

MYTHS ABOUT BULIMAREXIA

When we began our group work, we soon found that most women were eager to share their histories. It was as if they were trying to shock each other, to out do one painful story with another. At the same time, it was clear that they had certain misconceptions about their binge/purge behavior. The following are the most usual—and the most crucial:

1. *Bulimarexia is a disease, a mental illness.* To categorize this syndrome as a disease is dangerous. Many women who engage in this behavior would like to believe that a disease or illness has overtaken them. We are convinced that bulimarexia is a learned behavior—a *habit* that can prove exceedingly difficult to give up. However, if it is learned it can be unlearned, utilizing basic principles and techniques to be discussed in this chapter. Those who insist that the binge/purge syndrome is a disease run the

risk of believing that someone does "it" to them and someone must cure them. In any case, the "victim" is off the hook!

2. *It has taken years for me to become bulimarexic; therefore, it will take years to stop.* This self-defeating philosophy only results in a stronger commitment to a bulimarexic lifestyle. By clinging to such an attitude, the woman allows herself no chance to try other, possibly more productive behaviors. With help, most women can acknowledge the irrationality of this years-to-stop premise and develop more realistic alternatives to stress than bingeing. We often point out that women who have been chronic bingers for fifteen to twenty years have curtailed or eliminated the behavior in a few months. Women who have been successful are usually eager to share their experiences with others still engaged in the struggle. We use their valuable suggestions in our group by way of letters, tapes, and, whenever possible, direct involvement. In this way we can *show* rather than *tell* the struggling bulimarexic that her basic belief system is not only in error but is serving to hold her back.

3. *Unless I understand why I binge and purge, I'll never be able to give it up.* Although the pursuit of underlying causes is fascinating and occasionally rewarding, it has typically resulted in extreme frustration and failure for the vast majority of bulimarexics. In fact, their obsession with *why* they binge and purge consumes most of their valuable energy, leaving them especially vulnerable to continued failure. As an alternative, we invite them to abandon this elusive pursuit and join us in concentrating on *what they get* from gorging and purging. What are the payoffs? How is the behavior serving them? Is it really *helping* them to avoid pain, responsibility, and/or intimacy? Does the binge and purge actually serve to punish others or are they really defeating themselves over and over again? Since behavior is purposive, we emphasize that a person does not typically adhere to a particular behavior unless something is derived from it. Shifting the emphasis from *why* the woman is bingeing and purging to *what* reward the behavior is offering allows her to discover, often for the first time, *how* bulimarexia is serving her.

4. *If I'm to give up gorging and purgeing, I must do so on my own.* Such a belief, admirable as it may seem at first glance, has inhibited growth and development for countless bulimarexic women. Although self-reliance is in line with contemporary feminist psychology, it is inappropriate in this particular context. The bulimarexic woman, in the throes of her difficulties, quite simply is not capable of sustaining herself independently. She is, in fact, *most vulnerable* when she is alone! Thus, it makes little sense to ask her to rely exclusively upon her own resources. Since the bulimarexic rarely binges or purges in the presence of others, we strenuously encourage her to develop sources of support, often with other group members, and to set up goals (goal contracts) with these individuals. These contracts must be specific and easily evaluated on a regular basis. The people selected for support, the nature of the contract, and the way progress is assessed are crucial. For example, it is not enough for the woman simply to ask a friend to "be there when I need you." This is far too ambiguous a contract. Instead, when the bulimarexic feels that the person she has in mind is willing to offer support and capable of doing so, she must then check this out with that person. If the chosen friend is another bulimarexic, the contract must be initiated with care. Because of their pervasive people-pleasing tendency, most bulimarexics will try to help even when they feel overwhelmed and incapable. Thus it would be wise to assess the situation realistically before making an explicit contractual agreement. Furthermore, contracting with only *one* person is unwise. That person may not be available for support at that particular time, which may lead to an irresistible urge to binge. This can often be avoided by acknowledging the potential problem and developing flexible contracts with a few friends as backups.

It is important for the bulimarexic woman to be exact in informing her potential sources of support about *her specific needs.* Take the example of Karla, who had been living by herself for almost a year and who had a history of extreme bingeing alone in her

apartment, often for days. When she left the group, Karla had decided to call either Jenny, Laura, or Alice *only* when she had exhausted all of her own strategies to ward off bingeing. Weeks after
her experience in the group, Karla was faced with a number of
anxiety-arousing situations. After several unsuccessful attempts at
coping, she felt depleted and in need of support. Her first call
went unanswered; Jenny was out. In the past, this would have led
to a binge; however, because Karla had agreed to reach out to others, she immediately called Laura. This time she connected. But
Laura was having an argument with her husband, and since their
original contract was predicated on honest communication, she informed Karla that she could not deal with additional pressure at
that point. Laura asked Karla to call back the next morning.

Karla was frantic, yet she understood. Before calling Alice, she
decided to write down her feelings, to clarify what she needed at
this crucial time. The bottom line was reassurance about a painful
decision she had recently made to abandon a relationship with a
man that seemed to be going nowhere. The sense of isolation,
aloneness, and inadequacy that she was feeling terrified her. She
needed to feel connected to someone—or something. Reminding
herself that she was under considerable stress, Karla made an appointment at a local health spa instead of raiding the refrigerator.
Afterward she telephoned Jenny, who had returned home. They
met later, and Jenny, listening intently, genuinely reassured Karla
that she was right to end the relationship. Jenny also pointed out
that such a decision was not irreversible and could be reevaluated
at a later date. Most important, Jenny marveled at Karla's strength
and ingenuity in avoiding gorging under pressure. Thus both
women maintained an honest, supportive stance. Karla showed
herself and her friend that she could avoid bingeing and could
reach out for specific help even in extreme anxiety. In retrospect,
Karla realized that despite her attempts to cope, she had panicked
prematurely, reaching out before doing her "homework" and clarifying in writing what she felt she needed.

The next day Laura called Karla, having worked through her crisis with her husband. When Laura heard of Karla's success, she

was equally genuine in reinforcing her friend. There was no need for Laura to apologize for the previous evening since openness had been a condition of their contract.

It is unfair and potentially self-defeating for bulimarexics to ask for help and then expect others to know precisely how to respond. Relatives and close friends often feel that they were at least partially responsible for the initiation and/or maintenance of the woman's behavior, and their guilt and helplessness can make them reluctant to support her when she makes strides toward recovery. However, those closest to the bulimarexic need to feel that they are part of her success experiences and the ensuing recovery process. Unless they do, sabotage is likely even though not intended. This sabotage can be subtle, as in the case of Claire, who moved out of her parent's home and returned to report good progress only to find both parents unwilling to trust that the gains would be permanent. In other instances, damage can be more overt. Janie's husband insisted that she eat alone each evening in order to demonstrate that she was completely cured. During this time, Janie said that her husband was quite punitive and demanding, as if he were "invested in keeping me a prisoner to bulimarexia." Obviously, the husband's attitude was not helpful, but Janie had not indicated exactly what she expected of him.

5. *As a bulimarexic I am powerless in the face of food.* This assumption feeds directly into the bulimarexic's sense of learned helplessness. It is not only illogical, but it successfully prevents the woman from self-motivation. Fortunately, this is the easiest assumption to dispel. Former patients who have been chronic bingers and purgers and who have, within a few weeks or months, developed the capacity to enjoy a palatable meal prove that it can be done.

The sense of powerlessness so familiar to anorexics and bulimarexics is often reinforced by popular articles about eating disorders. An article in the *New York Times* a few years ago referred to anorexics as "victims of the disease." Another, in *People* magazine, carried the headline: "A Dangerous Eat-&-Purge Disorder Called Bulimia Strikes Young Women." Even more devastating was an article in *Time* magazine that indicated that "there were no known cures" for bulimia. Thus the language used to describe these syndromes can inadvertently heighten a despair that is already extreme.

6. *When I stop bingeing and purging, everything will be fine.* This naïve view either results in consistent disappointment and more frequent bingeing, or it lets the woman off the hook. There is no way that this expectation can be fulfilled. Furthermore, such a belief holds the *syndrome* accountable rather than the *person* who chooses to engage in binge/purge behavior. It is a not so subtle trick that the bulimarexic plays on herself and others. By maintaining that bulimarexia—that insidious, uncontrollable disease process—makes her life miserable—the woman makes a commitment to despair. To believe that life will be troublefree when she stops bingeing is an excellent way of insuring that bingeing will continue with a vengeance. After all, who among us is capable of controlling life so as to avoid discomfort completely? It is not coincidental that the bulimarexic often adheres to this myth, however. As mentioned earlier, she is a perfectionist interested in avoiding pain. And she will not allow herself even one mistake! She may be able to avoid bingeing for weeks or months, but *one mistake* usually results in a return to extreme binge/purge behavior.

She is really saying, "Unless I am guaranteed that my life will be troublefree when I stop bingeing and purging, I will not give it up." Many a bulimarexic has admitted to this with a twinkle in her eye! This is a good beginning, for unless she is capable of "owning" the behavior, there is little she can do about it.

INDIVIDUAL THERAPY WITHIN A GROUP CONTEXT

Although bulimarexic women are willing to identify with one another, they soon become aware that they are dissimilar in many ways. If such differences are not acknowledged, group disharmony can ensue. Group members may indicate that they do not feel "like everyone else here," claiming that their binges are not as severe, that their lifestyles are quite different, and that differences in age serve to separate them from other members. They are, of course, correct when they point out these differences. However, such observations in no way negate the therapy process. What is crucial, then, is to *individualize* the treatment program for each group participant. Unless each woman is allowed to feel her individuality as an asset, she may well resist help through therapy yet remain in the group. Her presence then becomes a deterrent to the process of change. If we can redirect attention toward common goals, considerable vicarious learning can take place.

Focusing on the "payoffs" derived from bulimarexia often serves to unite the group. For there are very few payoffs. In brief, gorging and purging come to be seen as either avoidance behaviors or as means of punishment. For some, it is the avoidance of intimacy, for others, the avoidance of success. Still others use bingeing and purging as a way of avoiding failure. Another contingent of bulimarexic women, particularly those in their late teens and early twenties, use bingeing and purging to elicit attention and punish parents and others. In many such cases, the family is well aware of the bulimarexia and may even watch helplessly while the woman binges. A young woman may binge in order to avoid the awesome pursuit of success and, at the same time, cause her parents, who have consistently urged her to do well in all she encounters, to feel guilty. Another woman, on the verge of success in school or in the work world, may return to severe bingeing out of fear of failure and, at the same time, punish her husband who, she feels, has not supported her in some important way.

When several group members have identified what maintains

their bingeing, they usually begin to identify with one another. Their sense of sisterhood and camaraderie is thus enhanced. It is not absolutely necessary for each woman to discover what she is deriving from her destructive behavior. Some are not ready to acknowledge this, some feel incapable of doing so, and others already know but have done nothing to effect change. Those who do know often begin to consider alternatives to bingeing. Those who do not can observe those who do. Later they too may be able to address this particular issue. It is especially important not to convey the notion that insight into the payoff is necessary before the basic binge/purge cycle can be altered. At least 25 percent of the women we have worked with never identified their payoffs within the group yet later were able to curtail or eliminate their binge/purge pattern on their own. Interviews with one hundred such women suggest that most of them (usually after the group experience) made major modifications in the way they adapted to life situations only to realize that the new behavior served them far better than bingeing. As might be expected, these women were generally less animated and verbal during our formal group therapy sessions.

REWRITING THE SCRIPT

Certain negative concepts make up the life script of the bulimarexic. A new understanding of the concept of *irreversibility* often helps to move women beyond their eating impasse. We emphasize that there are few behaviors that are irreversible and invite the women to explore new ways of dealing with their anxiety. We point out that their old ways do not appear to be working, so why not give some new ones a try? Unless the new ways are more palatable and productive, they always have the option of returning to bingeing. What we are asking for is a commitment to a new strategy. We caution the women that anything new will feel unfamiliar. The new and unfamiliar can be uncomfortable for any of us and particularly so for the bulimarexic.

Most bulimarexics will wholeheartedly agree that their old ways have not been helpful and are therefore willing to explore new means of coping with the stress and anxiety that characteristically lead to a binge. Such a commitment thereby forces them to confront two major deterrents to psychological growth that not only characterize the bulimarexic, but are frequently present in all of us.

In dealing with the stresses and anxieties that lead to bingeing, *the bulimarexic has learned to avoid pain at all costs.* If she is to change, she must learn to use painful thoughts as *motivators* rather than as excuses to binge. Pain is a precursor of change, particularly for those who are committed to gaining strength. Even a brief sojourn into our past will remind us that those experiences of which we are most proud can typically be traced to painful thoughts and acts that we used to motivate risk taking. We therefore emphasize the importance of reevaluating each woman's methods of coping with pain by helping her to identify and troubleshoot her avoidance patterns. For example, Shelley, a former athlete, had decided that instead of competing and risking the pain of losing, she would simply avoid competitive sports. Before long, she felt that she rarely enjoyed any activities with other people and claimed that she was bored and becoming more reclusive.

Shelley was persuaded to join a bowling team, a sport she had previously enjoyed until the team members urged her to compete for team captain. In retrospect, she admitted that even if she had been able to control her anxiety and deal with her rivals' bantering, she did not want to be captain. She was not ready for the limelight, despite her obvious skill as a bowler. Now, when she was asked to "rehearse for catastrophe," Shelley said that her greatest fear was that she would be judged adversely, especially by "expert bowlers." Actually, she was her own worst critic, constantly alluding to her imagined ineptitudes. Other group members soon helped her to see how she set herself up for ridicule—how she planted these thoughts in others. Shelley agreed to try to substitute more realistic messages to herself when she was bowling. Such statements as, "I know I'm going to blow it now," "This is an impossible spare," and "I'm sure Sarah will never forgive me if we don't win" were rephrased as "I'll give it my best now," "I'll try and pick up this spare by . . . ," and "Sarah seems so intent upon winning—I feel that pressure and am therefore going to *ask her* what she's feeling."

By ceasing to anticipate the worst, Shelley was able to enjoy healthy competition once more while satisfying her need to be gregarious, which had gone unfilled for nearly five years.

Most bulimarexics also live either in the past or in the future. When confronted by a situation that is moderately challenging, they look to the past for coping strategies (bingeing) or look ahead and rehearse for tragedy (nothing will work out). Since the past cannot be changed and the future is, for the most part, unpredictable (or contingent upon what one does in the moment), we encourage group members to replace these habits with a *present, action-oriented attitude.* The women learn to talk to themselves *in the moment* and to engage their "old" part and their "new" part in a dialogue at the moment pain begins. Such "top-dog/underdog" techniques forces an important dialogue that is first undertaken aloud in the group so that all can help the woman to deal with unsure and irrational beliefs that have reinforced top dog for so long.

By way of illustration, consider Diane, a "5 o'clock binger." Each afternoon after work, Diane headed straight for the supermarket. When she claimed that she was "magnetized by the place," we encouraged the pessimistic part of her (top dog) to indulge in this belief. Underdog was then invited to speak. The quality and intensity of this monologue was, at first, pathetic. Group members joined to bolster underdog and with time and support, Diane began to invest this neglected yet vital part of herself with more energy. She soon recognized that top-dog statements were based almost exclusively upon *past* and *future* considerations, whereas underdog was present oriented. Top-dog statements were loaded with "can'ts" and similar pessimistic beliefs based upon past failures, or they reflected expectations that were essentially unwarranted (*"Yes,* I could try that, *but* I doubt it will work"). Underdog statements ("I want to try an alternate route home") reflected new strategies that could be undertaken in the present. As such, they could be evaluated and, if necessary, troubleshot. Diane saw the irrationality of top dog and, with the help of the group, began to confront this element before succumbing to its toxic message. By the end of the group experience, Diane was reexamining her script and rewriting it. Underdog was gaining strength and was consistently reinforced by all of us. Thus unless the bulimarexic is willing to ask "What tense am I in?" (present rather than past or future) when confronted by anxiety-arousing stimuli, she will, more often than not, follow her old script and fail to grow.

Another stumbling block to change involves what we call the "bionic woman syndrome." Bulimarexics expect perfection. They may, for instance, remain binge-free for weeks, only to encounter problems that trigger overeating. After one lapse, rather than scrutinizing the setback and learning from it, they classically revert to full-fledged gorging and purging. What is important here is their unwillingness or inability to reward themselves for their obvious strength over a period of weeks and to profit from that single mistake by troubleshooting what led to overeating. Through "homework assignments" that involve specific scenarios that set the stage for a binge, the bulimarexic brings to the group a number of alternatives that can then be examined. Each woman thus rewrites her script in a trial and error fashion. Because *she* is the principal author, she often overcomes resistance to change and has more energy to devote to this valuable and rewarding pursuit. In Shelley's situation, homework logically followed from the role plays centering around bowling. In fact, upon leaving the group one evening, she and three group members engaged in a shuffleboard contest. All eyes were upon her, especially when game pressure was high. Although Shelley did poorly and lost a game for her team, she performed well in other ways. By self-monitoring her pessimistic statements and avoiding interpretation and analysis of the other women, she not only delighted in the excitement of the game but began to see how she could develop intimacy by sharing her feelings with her partner.

GOAL CONTRACTING

Each group member establishes her own goals, which she articulates in a specific fashion. She is now making an overt commitment in the presence of others with whom she has begun to feel comfortable. It is important at this point to clarify the difference between a *goal* and an *expectation.* Quite simply, an expectation implies an outcome. A goal does not; it merely represents a commitment to *try.* Since most bulimarexic women have defeated themselves countless times as a result of unrealistic expectations, we ask them to reassess this self-sabotage maneuver. Each woman reviews the most effective process she has employed to give up bingeing and purging. Invariably someone will describe a time when she was binge-free for weeks only to encounter real difficulties that precipitated a relapse. Upon discovering that their expectation was that they would *never* binge again, the women soon realize that such perfectionism assures failure in the long run. Statements like "I'll *never* binge again" or "I'm giving this up *forever"* can only hamper well-intentioned bulimarexics.

This is also true of negative expectations. For example, "I know as hard as I try I'll never be completely binge-free" is a commitment to failure. Not surprisingly, bulimarexic women often say: "I must gain total self-control"; "I will no longer feel anxious and vulnerable with men"; "I should establish friendships with women without ever being competitive and mistrustful"; and "I must understand why I binge and purge." How much better if these expectations become goals that can be restated as: "I want to learn *what* I am getting from allowing myself to binge and purge"; "I want to try to communicate in an honest, straightforward fashion, especially with men to whom I am attracted"; "I want to take more risks with friendship, especially with women whom I admire"; and "I want to focus on *how* bingeing and purging are serving me in a variety of contexts." Now they are beginning to think in terms of how, when, and where they might accomplish specific objectives.

There should be a *number* of alternatives rather than a single alternative to bingeing since no one behavior is powerful enough to

displace bingeing under stress. Again, the group process is helpful
because of the similarity between one woman's particular avoidance
pattern and those of other women. Through this problem-solving
approach, the woman who is less likely to verbalize can feel a part
of the group process. Even so, each woman must ultimately try
some alternative ways of coping. Outside the group, all group
members are aware of the other participants' specific contracts to
take risks with new behavior. As therapists, we summarize individual goals and encourage the women to act as facilitators for
each other. The time the women spend together doing "homework" in the evenings and throughout the day is therefore as therapeutic as the time spent in formal session. As did Shelley, many
women actively explore a number of alternatives and experience
the consequences directly. Those who participate in these exercises
often stimulate other, less motivated women toward their goals.

Tina, one of the onlookers in the shuffleboard incident, wrote
recently regarding her progress. Although she never admitted it
during our group work, she had always felt guilty about being athletic, especially when she competed with men to whom she was attracted. Feeling that all men would reject her if she won, she would
often hold back in order that they might excel. Shelley's new strategy had impressed Tina. She respected Shelley, and they became
friends. Upon returning home, after some deliberation, Tina called
a man who she liked and admired. They went skiing, and she really "went for it." Much to her delight, he was impressed. With
time, they became ski partners, friends, and, ultimately, lovers.
Tina kept in touch with Shelley, whom she occasionally used as a
"sounding board for my new strategies." Although her relationship
with this man eventually came to an end, Tina continued to perform to the best of her abilities. She recognized that certain men
might be alienated by her competence, but, more important, she
discovered that others found her irresistible! Tina is now married
and attending medical school. As she pointed out, "It only took
eleven months to beat bulimarexia after I began to be real rather
than ideal." Showing the bulimarexic that what she *does* determines her identity and ultimately her sense of self is far more ef-

fective than simply telling her. We therefore place great emphasis upon helping women to discover that *they are what they do,* not what they think and feel.

Bulimarexic women do not know how to say no. By saying yes when they really mean no, they accumulate sufficient justifications for a later binge. This binge is "OK" because they have paid their dues by being available and accommodating when, in fact, they were really overloaded. The binge thus serves as a reward for being dishonest and accepting responsibility that they know they do not wish to handle. In their view, an honest, straightforward statement such as "I'm unable to help right now," is simply not polite. It is not feminine! In short, to say no when you do not wish to engage in a particular activity is less desirable than possibly offending others and assuring a binge.

In this same vein, the majority of bulimarexics have trouble accepting a compliment. This is easily illustrated in the group, particularly when we, as therapists, offer positive feedback. Although this behavior is understandable in light of the bulimarexic's poor self-concept, the inability or unwillingness to be rewarded stunts psychological growth. The occasional dishonest transactions that these women allow themselves only set the stage for bingeing. Elaine was classic in this regard. Beautiful, talented, and successful, she was a master of the "Yes, but . . ." game. Offer her a genuine compliment, and she would say, "Yes, but look at how weak and pathetic I am." At first, group members were sympathetic and continued to point out Elaine's assets, but they grew more and more frustrated as she continued to deprecate herself. This was perhaps best illustrated when we invited Elaine to troubleshoot (identify self-sabotaging statements) in the following role-play between Bill and Marlene:

MARLENE   You don't like the way I'm dressed, do you?
BILL   Yes, I think you look great!
MARLENE   Come on, Bill, I know you think this skirt looks foolish.
BILL   It's not my favorite, but I think you look great tonight.

MARLENE   See, you're just trying to make me feel good!

BILL   I'm being honest with you, Marlene. You really look fine.

MARLENE   But not great—you can tell me; I know I don't look great, right?

BILL   Well, whatever you say, but I still feel that you look very nice and I'm hungry, so let's go to the dinner party.

MARLENE   Hold on, I want to change into something else. I can't stand going out when you don't like the way I'm dressed.

What is preventing Marlene from feeling good about herself? This was the question we asked. Now that she was outside the experience, Elaine could zero in on Marlene's self-defeating style. Others were also helpful, particularly during time outside the group, in pointing out Elaine's pervasive habit and refusing to reinforce it. After consistent exposure to honest feedback, Elaine altered her put-down messages to herself and began to acknowledge her good qualities. Several months later she accepted a modeling contract in order to obtain enough money to attend college and begin a career as a physical therapist. Before the group experience, she had refused to "use my looks and figure instead of my mind." Now that she has explored a creative compromise, Elaine is no longer so myopic. She still binges occasionally but has given up the major "racket" that led to regular binge/purge behavior, perpetuated a poor self-image, and gave her an opportunity to get off the hook.

REDEFINING FEMININITY

Once the toxic behaviors described above are exposed, group members directly confront the major precursors of binge/purge behavior. As women in our culture, they have unwittingly taken the posture of accommodation to its extreme. What follows is a redefinition of the feminine role.

At this point, Marlene work alone with the group. The issues addressed depend on the particular makeup of each group. When it is composed of younger women, struggles for independence and problems with parents are often crucial. Groups of older, married women and mothers present different topics for examination.

Because of their basically dishonest lifestyle, intimacy is rare among bulimarexics. Few have close female friends, and those who do feel intensely competitive and mistrustful of female companionship. One of the primary goals of this segment of treatment is to facilitate open communication. Encouraging women to like and respect others with similar problems often serves to enhance their self-esteem. This is particularly important for bulimarexic women since they tend to relinquish their power, particularly in the presence of men. To illustrate this point, Marlene will frequently draw from earlier interactions that took place when Bill was present. She demonstrates how group members almost invariably vied for the attention of the male therapist, even attributing change to *his* intervention. Many are, in effect, acting as though they are in dire need of being rescued. However, women must develop their own strengths and capacity for growth if they are to achieve a sense of self. Oneness must precede twoness. And there are golden opportunities available to every woman, thanks to feminist principles and awareness. Thus, one goal of our treatment involves encouraging strong feelings of sisterhood among group participants. Reactions from scores of women over the years suggest that such a bond can be therapeutic in and of itself. This sense of connectedness ensures a support structure that sustains the women during the initial difficult months after treatment.

As part of our treatment program, group participants from the same geographical area are asked to room together. In addition, they are encouraged to spend time together outside of the group. Those who report increased feelings of self-worth because they are able to help and encourage one another begin to demonstrate less reliance upon us, the therapists.

Most bulimarexics have few women in their lives they can admire. Part of Marlene's function with the group involves sharing her personal struggles with the same issues of self-worth, body image, and acceptability to men. Group members are often curious to know whether Marlene was herself a bulimarexic. Some women seize on the fact that she was not. Some even claim she cannot understand their problem and are reluctant to acknowledge her insights. By describing her own imperfections, Marlene counteracts the concept of "bionic woman" and helps to dispel the myth of perfectionism. Group members can relate to her as a professional woman with her own problems. The myth of uniqueness is also exposed when it becomes apparent that all of the women have shared common feelings, mistakes, and failures. This kind of communication often gives the women a powerful sense of hope. They become aware that a different kind of future is possible.

Bulimarexics traditionally believe that a man's love will transform their lives by relieving them of responsibility. Each woman is therefore asked to assess what heterosexual relationships have meant to her. Many discover that by relinquishing responsibility for decision making, they have not only undermined their self-concept, but have alienated the men with whom they were involved. Often, with the help of the group, these women are able to understand the anger, resentment, and disillusionment expressed by fathers, husbands, and boyfriends.

Louise is a prime example. In order to avoid criticism, she gradually turned over her responsibilities to other people, one by one. First, although she had a degree in mathematics, she stopped writing checks when her husband complained because of an occasional overdraft. Then she stopped helping her daughter with her homework, turning this responsibility over to her eighteen-year-old son. She even gave up her part-time job as an instructor of gymnastics after a youngster, known for her caustic tongue, made a disparaging remark to her. In the process of diminishing herself, Louise became physically inactive and resorted to bingeing and purging in hopes of retaining her figure. Her husband, son, and daughter, frustrated in their attempts to intervene in what they considered "menopausal depression," became more and more resentful of and angry with Louise, finally insisting that she commit herself to a psychiatric hospital. After two months she was discharged and referred to us.

Upon entering the group, Louise was initially treated with compassion by the other women. But soon they began to realize that they had trapped themselves and, at the therapist's suggestion, initiated a role play based upon Louise's description of her former lifestyle at home. Anger and resentment emerged, and Louise, for the first time, realized that her gradual isolation from the family had precipitated much of the unpleasantness. Louise realized that she had become bored and was particularly vulnerable to bingeing. Nevertheless, she felt inept and unsure of her most basic skills. In order to assess this view of herself, Louise was asked to prepare a "mini-lecture" involving basic concepts in geometry. It so happened that Regina, a college sophomore and a group member, was having difficulty in a math course and had brought her textbook along. The following morning, after about an hour's preparation, Louise gave her lecture and was magnificent! Even the dullest among us was able to follow her succinct, professional presentation. More importantly, Louise was proud of herself. This proved to be a new beginning for a woman who, two months previously, had been hospitalized. Contracts involving more assertive behavior were then initiated and tested within and outside the group and later at home with her husband, who was described as domineering and critical yet eager to save their marriage. Louise has begun to take back her power, but not without considerable struggle. At present, she is working on a master's degree, and she has been binge-free for over two years.

In addition to risk taking and assuming responsibility, issues involving sexuality are often primary during the all-women part of the group. Many of the women admit to being nonorgasmic despite the fact that they crave sexual contact. They anticipate intercourse with trepidation, feeling inadequate and incapable of satisfying their partners (or themselves). Major emphasis is therefore placed upon how to communicate and thereby build a good sexual partnership. The first step in this venture is to examine the self-loathing these women feel toward their bodies.

For bulimarexics, the pursuit of slimness is their raison d'être. A common fantasy is that their lives will change when they are *thin enough*. In dispelling this fantasy, showing beats telling once again. Women in the group who are slightly overweight quickly perceive that exceedingly slim and beautiful group members also feel worthless and unlovable. The women begin to see that *they*, not men, turn themselves into sexual objects through a narcissistic preoccupation with weight and appearance. As they share their perceptions of their bodies and hear comments about the distorted images, many veer toward a more realistic assessment of their physicalities.

Those who are slightly overweight no longer exaggerate their flaws, and those slightly underweight seem to accept the need to add weight in a gradual, healthy manner. Marlene encourages the women to engage in sports and other physical activities. Emphasis is thereby shifted from inactivity or compulsive attempts to rid the body of dreaded calories to deriving pleasure from one's body.

Much of this session involves goal contracting, some of which includes important issues concerning men that can be undertaken with Bill at a later point. For example, during a group session, Gloria disclosed that she had been faking orgasm for fear of offending or losing her boyfriend. She also believed there was something wrong with her because she required sustained clitoral stimulation to become sexually aroused. Because she made no effort to communicate her fears to her boyfriend, he had assumed that everything was all right. Group members were able to assure Gloria that she was not abnormal.

At first, Gloria was embarrassed to discuss her sexual feelings so openly. However, as the other women spoke up, Gloria relaxed and expressed a desire to confront this issue in the group. A contract was therefore initiated, and Gloria was asked to participate in an "empty-chair" exercise by imagining that her boyfriend was sitting in the chair. Gloria was then asked to try new ways of conversing about sex with him. This was exceedingly difficult for her. She stumbled and muddled, was incoherent at one point, and became frustrated again and again. Such "mistakes" were identified as typical by other group members, and Gloria eventually discovered what she wanted to say to her boyfriend. She found that she liked herself best when she got rid of "sweetsy pie" and was "straight and direct." She had discovered one of the great yet elusive payoffs associated with being authentic and real.

Gloria continued to work on this issue with Bill when he rejoined the group. Since her boyfriend was exceedingly controlling, Bill's dialogue with Gloria was deliberately macho in order to assess her proposed strategies in the face of stress. Gloria fared quite well under this "rough handling," which helped her to realize that she was not as fragile as she had believed and therefore *acted.* Such scenarios underline the importance of the all-women part of the group. Few of these issues would have been raised had a male been present.

Assertiveness training is central to our treatment because bulimarexics are eager to appease others and to avoid conflict at any cost. Unfortunately, this kind of behavior is generally approved of and considered socially acceptable: The woman who is agreeable and ameliorating is a "good" friend, wife, or daughter. In the long run, however, appeasement results in loss of self-esteem and suppressed anger. Again, we have a classic precursor of bingeing. It is our task as therapists to help women develop more appropriate coping skills. Parent-daughter issues, husband-wife transactions, and mother-child problems are therefore played out to develop more active and responsible alternatives to the old ways of handling conflicts. Each woman can then demonstrate and practice these new alternatives and learn to accept the validity of her own emotions. The following example illustrates the importance of assertiveness and helps to define what the term "assertion" really means.

Jennifer bitterly complained that she was unable to sustain relationships with men. What she wanted more than anything was an intimate relationship. Because she had never had intimacy with a man, she considered herself a failure. Over the years she found herself dissatisfied with men in one way or another and would typically end relationships in the initial stages. After listening carefully, group members noted that Jennifer had certain mistaken beliefs about the way women should act with men. For example, she obviously equated assertion with aggression and thought that nonassertion meant that she was being polite and considerate. In defending herself, Jennifer spoke repeatedly about "not wanting to hurt his feelings." Not surprisingly, Jennifer's encounters with men were distressingly repetitive. Because she was strikingly beautiful, men were attracted to her. When a man tried to find out if she was similarly attracted to him, she would typically encourage him (even if she did not care for the man), not wishing to "hurt him." Having received what he felt were assurances, the man would pursue her more actively. Jennifer would then begin to "turn off" and, at the same time, hate herself for her deception. However, she typically placed the blame on the man for "pushing her" and developed even more devious maneuvers to avoid other men. She invested an inordinate amount of time into such demoralizing encounters so that, in the end, most of the men felt deeply hurt and "taken." Jennifer felt increasingly guilty and concluded that she was incapable of intimacy with men.

Jennifer was asked to try to communicate her feelings in a role-play, with Bill acting the part of her current boyfriend. At first, Jennifer had great difficulty maintaining eye contact with Bill. She hunched her shoulders, covered her mouth with her hand, and displayed a variety of nervous, distracting gestures. Her speech pattern was hesitant, with many pauses, and she acted in a subservient, self-effacing manner. Group members commented on Jennifer's mannerisms and described how she seemed to them. Marlene then reenacted and exaggerated some of Jennifer's responses in an attempt to *show* her how she appeared to others. Next some of the other group members modeled several alternative ways of relating and gently prodded Jennifer to take some risks and try some new ways of responding on her own. This was difficult for her, but after two or three attempts she was more animated, alive, and self-confident. She admitted that, despite its unfamiliarity, "it felt good to be honest." A few group members and Bill spontaneously expressed delight and respect for Jennifer's behavior, and she began to see the benefits of assertiveness. After all, she hated herself for being dishonest and constantly put herself down for her lack of courage. Jennifer's work, however, had just begun. Later that evening, she practiced her new communication skills with a young man she met at a pub. She stumbled and was unsure of what to say and how to say it, but in the process she learned that she was not as fragile as she had supposed. About a year later, Jennifer wrote of the fun and friendships she was having with men. They found her openness refreshing and rare. Bolstered by these successes, she became more and more committed to risk taking rather than to helplessness.

Like Jennifer, few women will need to binge if they have more productive ways of identifying and satisfying their needs. They will no longer find it necessary to stuff themselves to ward off anger if they can acknowledge and express it more appropriately. The same applies to all forms of stress. Instead of bingeing as an escape from studying, a break in routine becomes possible. Instead of turning to food out of boredom and/or loneliness, women can acknowledge their loneliness and learn to socialize. Instead of bingeing to escape from uncomfortable situations, they can discover how to say no.

NEW STRATEGIES IN OLD SITUATIONS

The bulimarexic is typically most vulnerable to bingeing and purging when she is *alone*. As pointed out earlier, it is important for these women to avoid being alone, at difficult times and places or with people who invariably elicit anxiety. Many women are likely to binge on the job. They keep junk food concealed in their desks, cars, or other convenient places where the hoard is not readily detectable. They can cut down on or eliminate sneak bingeing if they make a deliberate effort not to be alone. Also, it is not possible to binge uncontrollably if there is nothing to consume. Thus, at the very least, the binger who is truly committed to alternatives will reach out to others for social reinforcement and get rid of her supply of "irresistible" food. One successful experience, of course, does not guarantee another. She may very well resort to bingeing at a later time or in another place. However, even if she does, a different sequence of events has taken place. If successful, she has eliminated bingeing during a specific time interval (e.g., when she is on the job) or in a particular place (her car) or when she is with a certain person (her slim neighbor), something she had thought she could *never* do. In addition, by trying new strategies in these extremely difficult situations, the woman shows herself that she is capable of coping.

Lest she rehearse for tragedy or sabotage herself by choosing to remember past failures (with the built-in assumption that she will fail again), we ask her to *reward herself* for every success. For instance, if she is avoiding bingeing at home, she should plan to do something she enjoys and can easily carry out. She might list five possibilities. For example, she might enjoy a hot tub, listen to her favorite CD, go to a movie or a play, or call someone to whom she truly enjoys talking. The list is endless once one begins to recognize how important it is to be nice to oneself *consistently* and at *appropriate* times. It is often helpful at this point in treatment to point to the irony of bingeing and purging—though the binger is obsessed with her body, she does little to take care of it! In fact, she is well on the way to damaging her health. Thus any new strategy should involve being gentle with herself, especially when she has genuinely been tried. With time and practice, many women are amazed at their progress.

What if the woman fails to keep to her goal contract and succumbs to a binge? Then she must be willing to try another strategy. But the bulimarexic is often quite myopic. She sees only one alternative to anxiety. After giving in to the binge, she immediately admits failure and compounds the error by grotesque gorging and purging. At a time when remaining rational and alert is absolutely crucial, she stops—surrendering to her emotions. In that moment the battle is lost!

She should ask herself what her alternatives are now that she has made a mistake? There are always alternatives. One, the most common, is to purge and reinitiate the cycle. Another is to binge and then *stop and reevaluate* (troubleshoot) precisely what went wrong. In fact, unless she can make this reassessment, it is quite likely that a similar sequence of events will soon lead to further binges. If the woman cannot determine what "red lights" she raced through, she can always return to her first alternative—the purge. But, we ask her, what does she have to lose by reversing the sequence so that troubleshooting precedes purging or bingeing yet again?

There is, however, still another alternative. She could binge and *reach out* for support. At this point in treatment, we ask everyone to consider the following problem: A woman who is doing quite well weeks after the termination of the group is telephoned by another group member who is the midst of a binge. The former, for any number of reasons, feels incapable of supporting the latter. What would *you* do? The group discusses the problem without our help, pitting their new knowledge and clearly stated goals against the familiar attraction to being accommodating. This enables us—and the women—to see who needs further individualized work and in what areas such work will be necessary. For example, those who feel compelled to help despite their apparent inability or reluctance to get too involved need to understand better how important it is to be an honest partner. Those who recognize that they cannot be all things to all people (yet have difficulty accepting this) need to reexamine how the bionic woman syndrome sets them up for feelings of inadequacy and self-doubt. Those who decline to help someone in real distress, because they are sure that the person really does not need help, will need to learn to avoid interpretation and analysis. Those who, despite genuine understanding, realize that they cannot be with a friend for good reason are in touch with the major issues. What they do will typically be decided in the moment, as it must be when a bulimarexic is under stress.

What is particularly important, however, is how the woman feels *after* she has responded to the plea for help. There is, of course, no one right way to respond, and she may later feel she could have done better. But if she does not make the attempt, she fails to confront the old habits that have not served her well.

Finally, unless the bulimarexic is willing to take the risk of trying out new strategies, she is likely to remain locked into her behavior. During all those years of people pleasing, bulimarexics appear to have forgotten—or in some cases never really learned—that psychological growth comes about through initiating change. Most of us, no matter how inhibited or conventional, struggle with two mutually incompatible desires. On the one hand, we crave predictability. It is easy to stay with the tried and true. We do not wish to appear the fool! On the other hand, we feel the need to change. How else can we feel accomplishment? If we are what we *do*, we must acknowledge that variety in our lives is a necessary precursor of psychological well-being. Although the consequences of risk taking certainly help to shape our lives, without the *process*, little learning can occur. With these thoughts in mind, what remains is to develop strategies based on well-conceived risks.

We have found it particularly helpful to remind our clients to pay careful attention to the bottom line. We ask, What is the worst that could happen if you engage in a particular alternative? If the outcome is potentially devastating, the proposed strategy may be too extreme or in need of revision. For example, Sally had been living at home and working as a waitress for several months, having left college abruptly after a series of extreme binge/purge episodes. Bored and ashamed, she had been avoiding other people. Her parents, although supportive, felt compelled to lecture her about her future and what she should be doing. In the course of our group, Sally established the following strategy: She would quit her job, move out of her parents' home, find her own apartment, and enroll in a program in nutritional science at a state university.

Sally knows that she feels inadequate as a waitress, that her parents are right about what she should be doing, and that if she is to succeed, she must do something that satisfies her. So far so good. Now let us look at the bottom line: What if she does not like the university program or does not do well? In either case, she has learned a great deal more than she could have had she remained a discontented waitress. Furthermore, if she does not like it, she is at least in a better position to determine what parts of the entire process she did not enjoy. In this particular case, living alone proved to be a major stumbling block. After a semester of daily bingeing at 4:00 P.M. when she was alone in her apartment, Sally took a further risk and found a roommate. She chose not to share her secret with this woman; however, they did agree to spend time together each afternoon studying. This was Sally's idea, proposed so that she could devote time to her studies at an hour of the day when she felt most vulnerable. The women studied together, and, under Sally's direction, both learned to reward themselves for their efforts by attending campus events, dating, and jogging. Soon, and for the first time, Sally was able to share her history with her roommate-friend. After that, she was able to laugh at the behavior she had so carefully concealed for six agonizing years. As she put it in a letter to us: "I now know that because I can laugh at bingeing, I no longer fear it and can deal with it whenever I wish." Napoleon put it another way when he said that those who fear being conquered are already doomed!

Each of the women with whom we work enters therapy with a varying amount of "unfinished business." Several hours in the group are therefore devoted to troubleshooting those hurdles that are often considered insurmountable. In an attempt to convey how we approach this important work, we would like to present one group member's script:

ANDREA'S days are all pretty much the same. Her morning ritual begins with checking her stomach for signs of bloating and jumping on the scale for the bad news. She will weigh herself at least five times during the day. Agonizing over how she might stave off a binge, Andrea thinks ahead to lunch, vacillating between promising herself that she will fast the entire day and deciding to eat just yogurt. She deals with her children first, getting them fed, dressed, and off to school. Andrea enjoys the bickering and activity. Mornings are generally happy times. Bingeing hasn't yet begun, and she vows that today will be different—although deep down she knows that it won't be.

After driving her four-year-old to preschool, she heads for the grocery store to replace the food she consumed yesterday. She chooses a different store each day because she is convinced that all the clerks know about her. Andrea buys food she knows the children will like, assuring herself that she is not going to eat such junk. For the rest of the morning, she involves herself with errands and volunteer activities in a frantic attempt to avoid being home, where bingeing is easiest.

Having gotten through the morning without bingeing, she collects her daughter from preschool and returns home to find beds unmade, laundry piled high, and breakfast dishes beckoning. Mildly hungry, Andrea decides to eat one cup of yogurt for lunch while fixing her daughter a sandwich. Hunger intensifies! She wants more! She sends her daughter outside to play. Aware that her house is a mess, that her friend is getting a new one that she will decorate beautifully because she is so artistic and well organized, Andrea begins with the cookies.

Initially, eating seems pleasant. The first cookie tastes good, as does her child's leftover sandwich. She decides to make several more sandwiches while consuming the remainder of the cookies. Out of control, the binge becomes unpleasant, messy, and painful. Andrea then consumes copious amounts of water, milk, and juice as she has learned that vomiting is easier when she drinks a lot. In addition to the sandwiches and cookies, she eats a pound of cheese and a jar of peanut butter—all bought that morning to last the week. By now she feels about to explode!

She rushes to the bathroom. Cramming her finger down her throat and vomiting has become as habitual as struggling not to think about the waste of food, her lack of discipline, and her inordinate shame. Moments later Andrea scours the toilet, brushes her teeth, and weighs herself to be sure that none of the dreaded food is detectable. Returning to the kitchen, she calls her little girl so that they can make cookies. Her son will soon be home from school, and she has devoured all the snack food. As she beats the batter and licks her fingers, a second binge is initiated. The freshly baked cookies have dwindled from two dozen to eight by the time her son arrives. Andrea continues to binge, purging about an hour later. Realizing that her husband will soon be home and that she has consumed most of their intended dinner, she runs to the grocery store. Writing her second check of the day, she blames her husband, who she is certain desires her to be a petite, pretty housewife and mother.

Andrea returns home under pressure to prepare dinner. By now she has lost patience and is screaming and yelling at her family. Dinner takes place in an atmosphere of chaos. The kids are happy to have Dad home, so Andrea is left alone to clean up. As she does so, she continues to consume the leftovers. When she purges, she runs the water in the bathroom sink so no one will hear her retching. Vomiting is now quite painful; her throat is on fire, and the skin around her mouth is raw.

Her husband goes to bed at 10:00 P.M., suggesting that she do the same. Andrea feels too dirty and disgusting to make love and fails to understand how he could ever desire her, so she consumes a handful of laxatives to assure that all food will be removed. She watches TV for an hour, then joins her sleeping mate. At 3:00 A.M., as usual, she awakens feeling ravenous and ready to reinitiate the destructive cycle.

The past eight years have been a variation on this theme. Eating and obsessing about food have occupied an inordinate amount of Andrea's time. When she is not preoccupied with bingeing, Andrea pores through countless books on nutrition, dieting, and the psychology of self-help. She has also developed a reputation as a gourmet cook and superb hostess.

ALL members of the group listened intently to Andrea's story and took notes at our insistence. We encouraged them to identify the specific behaviors that precipitated Andrea's bingeing and purging and to help her troubleshoot these hurdles by concentrating on the way she chose to begin her day. Upon awakening, she immediately weighed herself, anticipating bad news. What purpose does this serve? If she recognizes this as a good example of rehearsing for tragedy, what alternatives does she have to call upon? At this point Andrea was placed on the hot seat. After considerable thought, she concluded that she did not have to weigh herself, indicating that she could instead go to her favorite room—the study—and begin to plan her day. Such an alternative was in no way unique. Andrea, as well as other group members, had used a similar strategy in situations of more obvious stress.

However, one alternative strategy, no matter how creative or exceptional, is seldom sufficient. The bulimarexic woman needs at least one further alternative as a backup. The challenges of day-to-day living are rarely mastered with one strategy. Not only does evaluating alternatives stimulate thinking at a crucial time, it also serves as a bulwark against additional threat.

Another alternative involved getting rid of the bathroom scale. This was easy since Andrea was the sole observer of its daily bad news anyway. Knowing herself and her tendency to function best in structured situations, Andrea modified this alternative somewhat. Like many bulimarexics, she fondly spoke of the "good-old days." At one time she had been an avid tennis player, but she left the club because of her fear of food and disdain for those who idled away their lives around the courts. Getting rid of the scale and adding an early-morning tennis match as a new activity therefore served as her second alternative. Her husband, Hal, played regularly, and she was still asked to play tennis by women friends whose company she used to enjoy. Furthermore, with the new indoor courts, foul weather could not serve as an excuse not to play.

Moving on, Andrea focused upon the volunteer work she had undertaken in hopes of avoiding bingeing. Honest evaluation suggested that the volunteer work had created unlimited opportunities to binge. Since she never really enjoyed this work, she did it poorly, feeling guilty about her lack of interest. Other more dedicated and competent volunteers, who occasionally censured her, compounded Andrea's guilt, which gave her a further incentive to engage in bingeing. Upon reminding herself that a person is what he or she does, Andrea concluded that she had been an unfulfilled wife and mother in many regards. She therefore decided to set new goals. She would plan daily afternoon activities away from home with her daughter. Her son, Billy, could also be involved. After all, home had become her major setting for gorging and purging. At this point a group member pointed out that someone had to make the bed, clean the house, and prepare the meals. Acknowledging this, Andrea again assumed responsibility. Aware that she was viewed as a woman of leisure because she had a master's degree and a lawyer husband who did not expect her to work, she felt that she should at least take care of her home. Nevertheless, she abhorred doing so. What were her alternatives? This time, Andrea quickly delineated three. First, she could do the work and then reward herself for having done so; along the way, she might also learn to accept strokes from others. Second, she could look for a part-time job and use some of the money to hire a maid. Finally, she could ask her children to help with the housework, thereby interacting with them in a more appropriate and rewarding way than she had before (i.e., as a model of cleanliness and discipline rather than as a person who is out of control and inconsistent) while teaching them how to clean and care for themselves and their surroundings.

Group members are usually excited and encouraged by the ease with which they help each other to generate alternatives. The process by which active strategies are arrived at is often contagious and may carry over to more realistic settings outside of the group. Evening homework assignments are designed to further elicit new responses to old situations. Because of the group's commitment to change, it soon becomes apparent that new habits can be substituted for old ones. What's more, as they pinpoint specific stimuli that bring on bingeing, many women discover that what is necessary is a *relabeling* of the situation rather than a reliance upon new strategies. Labeling themselves as "aroused" or "excited" instead of as "hysterical" or "anxiety ridden" allows them to *plan* rather than *retreat.*

After a few success experiences based on relabeling, most women see the benefits of this new way of responding. Troubleshooting strategies then may require further evaluation, but evaluation must now occur in an active realm. The women are likely to sabotage themselves if they try to think through each and every alternative, for we have found that bulimarexics can think themselves into or out of anything! This is the time for action. Whether various strategies can be easily integrated into daily life and whether relatives and friends will be sympathetic cannot be determined with certainty in advance. Each woman must therefore *react without expectation* once she has developed her alternatives. The worst that might happen is that she will not succeed. However, in the process, it is possible that she might discover, on her own or with the help of others, what led to a particular unsuccessful outcome.

Andrea had an experience that she spontaneously shared with the group. She felt that her sex life had been less than adequate ever since Hal and she had dated in college. She blamed this on bulimarexia. One night, in desperation, she decided to create a romantic setting in which to entertain Hal when he returned home that evening from a business trip. She sent the children to her mother's house for the night, dressed provocatively, chilled a bottle of wine, prepared an elegant meal, and awaited Hal's arrival by candlelight. When he arrived, he was overwhelmed by the reception. They made love magnificently, and Andrea remembered that evening for weeks thereafter. However, the pleasure of the occasion was not duplicated.

Andrea now revealed that it was primarily because of her expectations and lack of honest communication that she did not follow up on her sexual enjoyment with Hal. The problem was that she expected Hal to do something similar—and soon! After all, it was his turn, wasn't it? When he did not, she was sure it was because she was unattractive to him. Instead of communicating honestly with her husband, she assumed her interpretation was accurate and resumed her nightly bingeing and purging. Hal's attempts to initiate further sexual involvement were thereby thwarted.

Realizing that she wanted a more fulfilling sexual experience with her husband, Andrea formulated new strategies. She decided to make a pact with herself. From now on she would *ask rather than interpret!* To begin with, she would attempt to initiate sexual encounters with Hal and encourage him to do so with her as well. Since she enjoyed being "social chairman," why not capitalize on this talent? In the next few months, Andrea found that she could effect significant changes in her sex life that carried over to married life in general. Much to her delight, Hal spent more time at home, and, with the help of a therapist, they began a new relationship based upon honesty and risk taking. Andrea occasionally overeats, but she no longer turns these infrequent lapses into extended binge/purge episodes. She has neither the time nor the inclination.

ALTHOUGH we had not originally intended it, our relationship as a couple often serves as a focal point for group discussion, since we tend to interact openly with one another. When we disagree before the group, our actions and words are often scrutinized in light of those crucial issues that are typically raised during the all-women session. Many of the fantasies and erroneous expectations that women attribute to men are thereby exposed. For example, most bulimarexics are convinced that men prefer to direct and teach women. Thus, when Marlene shows Bill where he is remiss, his response and her way of relating to him can be experienced directly. Quite spontaneously, we illustrate a variety of communicative skills that are foreign to many group members. In revealing our own struggles and deficiencies, we also help dispel the myth of the "perfect couple" and give the women another chance to evaluate and formulate new approaches to change.

Therapists are not immune to maladaptive behavior and can also profit from the suggestions of the group. Thus, the group process has something to offer everyone.

8 .

Intensive Psychotherapy with Bulimarexics

OUR original workshops were designed as psychoeducational, strategic-planning programs for bulimarexics and interested therapists who wanted to experience our work directly. We never meant them to be "definitive" treatment programs. Our goal was to share what we had learned from our clients; their effective strategies became the focus of these treatment workshops. Goal-contracting was tailored to the individual and the situation, but bingeing and purging were the primary issues addressed.

We found that few bulimarexics were able to "go cold turkey" and never binge and purge again. This was precisely what we expected. It was heartening, however, to discover that the majority of the women were able to *curtail significantly* their binge/purge behavior following an intensive fifteen-hour seminar.

After attending our workshops, many women sought further therapy, either returning to former therapists or seeking new ones. They were more assertive now, aware of the negative effects of viewing themselves as disease victims, and no longer convinced of their own weakness or stupidity. They could look for the kind of therapy they wanted and delineate goals to fit their present needs. At the same time, they were in a position to benefit from more traditional forms of therapy. It seems that most bulimarexics will not respond to insight-oriented therapy unless and *until* they can attenuate their binge/purge ritual. Once they are helped to do so, they are much more open to addressing and changing other aspects of their lives.

Eleven years later, we continue to offer weekend workshops. However, whenever possible we prefer to involve women in more intensive and consistent treatment.

INDIVIDUAL PSYCHOTHERAPY

One-to-one work with bulimarexics usually requires six months to a year. Generally, there is some attenuation of binge/purge behavior after one to three months of therapy, though lapses can be expected. The women learn that they can fail, troubleshoot, and fail again and again, but eventually they are able to adopt new strategies in old situations. Most of the women we see now have one hour of individual therapy a week and one hour of group therapy. By the end of six months, binge/purge frequency has been reduced from one to ten times daily to five to ten times a month.

The group experience then becomes the major means of treatment and may continue at least another six months. The gradual reduction of bingeing and purging is directly related to coping strategies and reinforcement of newfound strengths. Soon the women think of themselves as strong women who handle themselves with dignity under stress. Some can stop themselves in the middle of a binge session, while others are able to consume considerably less food than before. More important, *attitudes* about bingeing and purging are drastically modified. Lapses are now seen as opportunities to reevaluate behavior, learn, and grow. Let us now examine the process in detail.

The First Individual Session

The first one-to-one session with a bulimarexic is exciting and challenging. As therapists getting acquainted with a dynamic and engaging young woman, we like to obtain as much personal history as possible. This includes a detailed history of eating behavior. It is important to know also whether the client was ever overweight or underweight. What were her highest and lowest adult weights? How and when did they occur and how long were they maintained? What was a woman's eating pattern before she became bulimarexic? What was going on in her life at the onset of eating problems? How intense is bingeing and purging now? How long, and how frequent? What types of food and amounts are ingested during a binge? Where does the woman engage in binge eating? Who knows about this behavior?

The method or methods of purging are important to understand too. If laxatives, diuretics, or amphetamines are used, what is the frequency of use, the type and dosage? How much exercise does a woman engage in? Is she menstruating? Does she have mood swings? Does she sleep well? Does she abuse alcohol, cocaine, or other drugs? What about the rest of her life at work, at school, and in relationships?

After gathering this history, we evaluate readiness to enter psychotherapy by discussing a number of essential factors in overcoming bulimarexia. Clients rate themselves on a scale of from 1 to 10, and we then contract to work with each woman on the area(s) of greatest weakness. Most require some help in all of the following:

Commitment: The degree of commitment to overcoming bulimarexia is almost always related to the degree of pain the client is experiencing when she comes to therapy. Typically, something is on the line. A boss is saying: "I don't know what your problem is, but you've been absent too much. You're going to lose your job!"; a parent is saying: "I'm not going to subsidize your habit anymore. You're on your own!"; a valued relationship has been terminated or weakened; a woman becomes pregnant or physically ill. Frequently, a client is not motivated to change her behavior. When this is the case, it is important for a therapist to be honest and tell the woman that the prognosis is poor.

Terri, a nationally known celebrity, decided to take time out from her busy schedule to "get cured," as she put it. During the first therapy session, she giggled frequently. It soon became clear that she saw no good reason to give up bingeing and purging. She was highly successful in all aspects of her life, and three men said they loved her in spite of her bulimarexia. After the session, we suggested that Terri return when she felt motivated to work. Terri did return two years later, admitting that she had been reluctant to change her behavior until now. She had been dismissed recently from a film set because of chronic tardiness, due, of course, to bulimarexia, and was ready to work in earnest. This time we accepted her willingly. Years of disappointment have helped us to realize that it is a waste of time, energy, and money to work with clients who do not have a high commitment to change.

Courage: Alfred Adler has revealed how depression is a problem of courage, developing in people who are afraid of life and dependent on others. In Adler's view, these people live lives of "systematic self-restriction": The less they do on their own behalf, the less they can do and the more helpless and dependent they become. The more they shrink back from the vicissitudes and adventures of life, the more inept they feel.

To eliminate binge and purge behavior without helping the client with new, self-enhancing coping *strategies* is irresponsible and dangerous. Since bingeing, for most women, is a way of avoiding discomfort, initial attempts to attenuate the behavior are accompanied by feelings of loneliness, emptiness, and pain. During this time, clients need supportive therapy. Women report strange mood shifts as they no longer rely on bingeing to render themselves "unconscious" under stress. Angry flare-ups can occur. The little mouse begins to roar! The people pleaser snaps and snarls. Some parents have said that they wanted their "good girl" back—and sometimes she returns.

An additional problem during this period is that every new behavior feels uncomfortable, even phony. The old accustomed stress reducers are no longer sanctioned. A woman's courage needs to be consistently supported. Anxiety has become a powerful *demotivator.* So sensitized to feeling anxiety that they rarely examine the bottom line, such clients must learn that anxiety can be a powerful and essential response to threats. They need to restructure their thinking and reevaluate and relabel rather than panic and retreat. For example: "Oh, my God!" can become "Oh, wow!"

We often tell clients the story of two women crossing the railroad tracks. One is bulimarexic and the other is not. Both women get stuck in the tracks. Off in the distance they hear the train approaching. Immediately and habitually, the bulimarexic throws herself before the oncoming train, helpless and without hope in the face of threat. Her nonbulimarexic sister, thrashing and fighting, refuses to believe she is unable to free herself and manages to do so.

So we ask the bulimarexic to react courageously even though she does not feel secure. We remind our clients of Adler's belief that there is only one important difference between normal and neurotic individuals: Both *feel* little and small, but the neurotic *acts* it! Since any new behavior will feel unfamiliar, commitment, practice, accepting lapses, and troubleshooting are essential to overcoming a fear of failure (or success).

Discipline: We do not subscribe to the view that bulimarexia is a disorder of maturation—or a breakdown in the transition to adulthood, one theory presently in vogue. On the contrary, it seems to us that many of our clients are *too* responsible in many aspects of their lives. They are compulsive, orderly, and disciplined in their work routine and very particular about appearance. We often point out how carefully they have dressed for their session. The women we see seldom present a dismal, pathetic picture, and typically they have experienced considerable success.

The inability to overcome bulimarexia is often their first major failure. Although they try admirably *on their own* to eliminate bingeing and purging, they are seldom able to sustain the change because their expectations are too high. Unfortunately, they have been hunting elephants with BB guns! The dilemma is as follows: Bulimarexics feel stressed, in pain, or uncomfortable, feelings common to all of us. However, instead of asking themselves: "What do I need now?" they automatically respond with a binge, which assures that they will feel worse about themselves and weaker when faced with the stimuli that triggered their maladaptive response. The

problem lies in their response to stress. When they binge and rehearse for tragedy, the stress continues to mount. Over time and
through lack of practice, their adaptive skills become rusty, and
they cease to grow. The major task, then, is to help clients apply
their skills at discipline to stress management and food. For most
women, it is simply a matter of generalizing skills they already have.

FOOD FOR THOUGHT

During the first therapy sessions, it is important to emphasize certain facts about bulimarexic behavior. Most women started the behavior because they expected it to be effective in weight control.
Actually, bingeing and purging is an extremely *poor* way to *control*
weight. There is sufficient evidence that in a very short time the
women will begin to gain weight in spite of intensified purging. A
number of researchers have begun to observe this phenomenon.
Women who purge are suffering the consequences of lowered metabolism and are at starvation level most of the time. As a result,
the biological mechanism of binge eating is set in motion. What
these women need is help in developing sensible eating patterns—
with emphasis on *restrained consumption, not dieting*—while they
are attempting to cut down the frequency of purging. Some of our
colleagues insist that clients follow a specific food plan. Initially in
our treatment efforts, we believed that discussing food intake was
diversionary. We now know this thinking was shortsighted. It *is*
important to consider food consumption and diet. We now ask
clients to record their food intake carefully for a week. We discuss
the metabolic disturbances that have occurred and the assumptions that exacerbate their fears of being fat. Many women believe
they will gain weight if they consume more than six hundred calories a day! This *may* be true for some women *when bingeing and
purging*. It seems to take from three to four months without
episodes of purging before normal metabolic function is restored.
Well over half of our clients lose weight once they are able to ame-
liorate bingeing and purging in a significant way.

Clients who enter therapy wish that a fairy godmother could grant them three wishes: (1) to stop bingeing and purging; (2) to lose weight; (3) to never have to *think* about food. We tell them that therapy can deliver on the first and perhaps the second wish. However, it's unlikely they can stop thinking ("forget") about food. Surveys of women who are not bulimarexic seem to show that they maintain slimness by allowing themselves a three- to four-pound weight fluctuation. When they reach their upper limit, food consumption is *cut down*, not out. At the upper limit they also increase exercise. Feelings of anxiety are thereby controlled. With regard to exercise, about half of our clients are compulsive exercisers; the other half rarely exercise, and it's exceedingly difficult to motivate them. Week after week they come up with "yes, buts" but do little. The power of the group is the most effective motivational strategy as exercisers begin to encourage their lethargic sisters and, with our help, eventually make contracts with one another. Once they begin to exercise, little encouragement is required as fat becomes muscle and interest in aerobics becomes the alternative to planned and unplanned bingeing.

The Rules and Goals of Therapy

Clients are expected to participate in at least three months of individual psychotherapy and concurrent group treatment on a weekly basis. Those who break appointments are charged for the session unless they give us twenty-four-hour notice. When a parent or insurance company is underwriting the cost, as is the case with many college students, it is easy to be delinquent, especially when things are not going well.

We involve the family whenever possible. Even though parents may live hundreds of miles away, we try to make them part of the healing process and encourage visits to them and from them. It's useful to prepare parents before a client returns home lest they unwittingly reinforce maladaptive behavior. We explain that the best interventions are those that involve the client in the decision-making process. Nearly all of our clients opt to involve parents in the treatment process once they are convinced of the advantages.

The following goals are central in our treatment with clients and close relatives: We insist that bulimarexic behavior be attenuated slowly and gradually and discourage cold-turkey strategies. Although many of our clients can curtail binge/purge behavior for days at a time, most don't know *how* they did it and are likely to experience more frequent lapses. We stress the importance of not making the same mistakes over and over again. Good therapy involves turning big mistakes into little mistakes by consistent troubleshooting. Finally, clients must agree to try—from this day forth—at least three different alternative behaviors before bingeing. The binge then functions as a reward for having tried and troubleshot alternatives instead of simply as an excuse.

The alternative strategies for each client should be articulated and practiced inside and outside of treatment. As therapy sessions progress, the client reports what strategy she tried or will try. The therapists and group members pinpoint possible areas of sabotage and pose various situations for clients to handle. For example, should June's first strategy when she feels like bingeing at 4:00 P.M. be jogging? Never having jogged before, she goes out and buys a jogging suit and shoes. Wearing $150 worth of new clothes, she decides to jog a couple of miles the first day. Two hundred yards down the road she already hates jogging! She reminds herself of all the money she has spent, and as others streak by, she convinces herself once again that she is hopeless. She binges at 4:30, after her "jog." Even though she has "failed," this client's behavior is far better than it has been since she delayed a binge. In working through this dilemma, the client might be encouraged to walk two miles each day for the first week, gradually increasing the amount of exercise.

Homework is often generated for the next therapy session. Clients are usually asked to bring a list of "red-light" situations, with the most difficult people, places, and events that typically precipitate binge eating at the top, followed by less threatening situations. Women soon begin keeping a record of binge eating and purging episodes, the *time, place,* and *specific circumstances* of these binge/purge episodes, the *kinds* and *amounts* of food consumed, and their feelings *before, during,* and *after* a binge. Where did the binge occur and with whom, if anyone? We are interested to know if women felt like bingeing and purging but did not. Most bulimarexics, as they begin to attenuate the behavior, tend to emphasize their "mistakes" and ignore their successes. We want to know about the binges they *staved off.* Bulimarexics typically fail to take responsibility for their mistakes—"it is the demon, the force, magic, or someone else" who caused them to binge. By the same token, they do not take responsibility for their successes, even maintaining they are at a loss as to how they did so. We insist that they reward themselves when rewards are appropriate.

Homework Tips

Here is "homework" generated by a recent client that is particularly well thought out and impressive. She utilizes a simple "Shut up!" as a thought interruption strategy.

STRATEGIES TO STOP EATING SO MUCH:
Don't be alone! (1) Leave the house; go anywhere where you will be near people. If you want to be home, (2) don't check the cabinets—don't even go into the kitchen if you can help it, (3) call a friend—Mom, Dad, old friends from home, (4) check your e-mail, (5) play solitaire. Don't be afraid and don't feel like just because you are alone, you have to eat. You don't—that is no excuse to eat! If you want to eat when you are alone, do not get in the car. It is better to stay put, or if you go somewhere, do not take any money (meaning no bank card, checks, or cash allowed). Don't even carry money to school during classes—it's dangerous (especially change). Stay away from vending machines. (6) Tell yourself to "Shut Up!!"

FEELING HUNGRY BUT NOT WANTING TO EAT:
(1) Ask yourself, "Am I really hungry? When did you last eat? How many hours ago?" (2) Wait twelve minutes to see if hunger goes away. If it is time for you to eat and you really are hungry, eat around people at a table. Taste what you are eating. Realize it is fuel, not something to do,

and stop when you are done. Don't give up on yourself. If you shouldn't eat, (3) entertain yourself in any way, (4) go to the math emporium, (5) hang out with roommates, (6) take a bath, (7) read eating-disorder books, (8) drink water.

FEELING OF RESTLESSNESS.
(1) Relax by taking a bath, (2) play with your hair, (3) study. Think of the many other things in life besides food. (4) Go exercise if you feel the need to be doing something at all times—exercise takes a lot of energy. (5) If you are tired or bored, take a nap. If you aren't tired, try reading.

MOUTH FETISH:
(1) Call a friend if you need to be doing something with your mouth. Talking is a good substitute for food because its hard to talk and eat at the same time.

FINISHED WITH CLASSES FOR THE DAY:
(1) Don't go home straight to the kitchen. Bring lunch with you, and stay on campus to study. This way you are around people while you are eating. (2) Eat when your roommates are home. If they aren't home, don't eat unless you go where people are. (3) Decide a time that you have to be somewhere. Give yourself only a half hour to be home—go to the gym right after you eat lunch.

STRATEGIES FOR RED LIGHTS IN THE CAR:
(1) If you go out in your car, don't bring money unless it's for something specific (to pay a bill or enough money to buy only a diet soda). (2) go to exactly where you have to go, and then when you are going home don't make any extra stops. Tell yourself, "No, I am not going to stop anywhere—I don't need to." (3) Don't allow food into your car from this day forward. (4) Say, "Shut up! You are stronger than this!" (7) Think about if anyone saw you driving and eating—what a PIG!!

GOING OUT TO EAT:
Always order healthy meals (salads, chicken, substantial foods). Make sure it is going to fill you up. Make sure it is a real meal.

STUDYING:
You think it's hard to concentrate. Well, if you are eating, it takes the place of studying. You don't know how to do both at once. (1) Think how important school is to you. (2) Go to a place like the math emporium where

you aren't allowed to eat. (3) Again using "Shut up," remind yourself that school (getting a good grade on this test) is more important than food right now—you can eat tomorrow. You wake up better on an empty stomach.

NIGHTTIME:
Cut yourself off at 10:00 P.M. No eating after 10:00. You can do it! This way you will not have all the midnight snacks. This is the time of day when the most calories are consumed.

THERAPY IN PROGRESS

A good part of each session is spent looking closely at immediate progress and problems encountered during the past week. A client may discuss what she has learned from each mistake and what she will do the next time under similar circumstances. It is important to urge her to examine what could possibly interfere with this plan. One of our colleagues keeps a weekly chart of her clients' binge/purge episodes. She does not tell her clients she is doing this but will openly consult the chart to illustrate a point, since the perfectionism of the bulimarexic constantly interferes with her valid assessment of progress. Therefore, it is often helpful for a therapist to wait until a client is complaining about results to show her, on paper, that she has improved dramatically.

Another important aspect of the session is rehearsal for the following week. What problems might occur? What could throw the client for a loop? Such questions troubleshoot areas of stress and help clients refine strategies that foster more adaptive functioning. What bulimarexics really need is simple and clear and perhaps best illustrated by a case example. Jamie, a high school senior, had been struggling with eating disorders for many years before beginning therapy and attending our group. Hospitalized for anorexia, she had been diagnosed as a borderline personality. For three years she had been taking antipsychotics and antidepressants. Her diagnosis became her identity. For years the family had feared the loss of their daughter. Pitter-pattering around her, they had inadvertently catered to her weaknesses, temper tantrums, and breakdowns. When she entered therapy, years of helplessness, hopelessness, and reliance upon prescription drugs had negatively affected important areas of growth and development. She was exceedingly dependent on others and cried constantly. With the help of the group and intensive one-to-one psychotherapy, Jamie began to blossom after approximately two months. During a group meeting, as she described her recent successes and sobbed, this time for joy, she kept saying: *"I never knew I was supposed to be strong!"* This thinking was by no means unique. Questioning of the other women revealed that each of them had similar feelings.

Here are some areas of stress where women in general and bulimarexics in particular need help. These are the recurrent themes that appear in therapy; they are also the target of therapy.

Dealing with Unstructured Time Alone

Such a simple problem and yet so difficult for most women! We believe that this inability to be alone is related to the socialization of women. Our society has trained women *too well* in their role as caretaker. As a result, *few women know how to take care of themselves.* The right to relax, for example, is rarely seen as a right. Time out, if it occurs at all, is rehearsing for calamity, not refueling. It is not accidental that most bingeing and purging occurs at the end of the day, after a woman has carried out her major responsibilities in a competent manner. The college student binges at four o'clock in the afternoon after attending all of her classes. The working woman spends all day listening to the complaints of others and after work streaks to the nearest deli to give herself a break.

We ask our clients to supply us with a list of five reinforcers— situations, events, or people that bring them pleasure. Many women are stumped by this request. Few can come up with more than one or two pleasing situations. Therapy must therefore help women learn to reward themselves by taking time out for self-refreshment. College students who use bingeing as a delay tactic against studying or writing a paper need help with test anxiety and time management techniques followed by reinforcing breaks. The astute therapist urges work *followed by* reward—the horse before the cart. We encourage anything that will enhance the environment: painting a room, hanging pictures, creating a personal space. These strategies can also be beneficial for the homemaker who binges on the nights her husband is away from home. We also emphasize personal rituals that are pleasing such as giving oneself a facial, manicure, sauna, and so forth. Until women take care of themselves, others are not likely to do so.

Ironically, the only "breaks" some women take are exercise breaks. Although exercise is often therapeutic, it might not be playful, an experience the bulimarexic needs (allowing the child within some enjoyment).

Bulimarexics invariably use boredom as an excuse to binge. We point out that boredom can be overcome by goalcontracting. We ask clients what action they are going to try and pin them down by asking them to outline how, when, where, and with whom they will accomplish that action. We keep a close watch for evidence of sabotage. Session by session, clients are encouraged to take *action* and further encouraged when they do. Movement in the right direction deserves a twenty-one-gun salute.

Oneness before Twoness

When it comes to relationships with men, most of the women we work with are unable to conceptualize themselves in the following ways: as a model and teacher for men; as a partner in the *most* responsible manner; as being *completely* honest with men—i.e., real instead of ideal; as saying no to men; and so on. What these women need is consciousness raising—they need to learn more about men and to develop friendships with men instead of engaging in the unrelenting pursuit of a relationship. A woman named

Hope provides a good example. She had gone steady all through high school. In reality, she had "known" only one man by the time she reached college. Her basic information about men was distorted by the fact that her steady adored her and gave in to her every whim. By the time she reached college, she had a rather grandiose perception of herself but no real care of self underneath. During her freshman year, she met many new men, and they began to pursue her. She broke up with her boyfriend and began to date other men. Much to her dismay, the new suitors rarely called back after the first date!

Hope's self-concept was soon shattered. She began to binge and purge, lost a great deal of weight, began to miss classes, and ultimately stopped seeing friends. Upon entering therapy, the following points were emphasized: Would she want to be with someone who didn't want to be with her? What happened when the men failed to call again? It turned out that she always *expected* the worst, so when something went wrong she blamed some flaw in her own character. We examined other possibilities. Perhaps Hope's straightforward, honest manner turned men away—but since this was one aspect of her personality she valued, we encouraged her not to hang on to the men who felt threatened. Over time, Hope began to treat men more realistically as equals. She joined a sorority and developed close women friends with whom she was able to spend a Saturday night *without bingeing*. Before long, men were attracted to Hope and began to confide in her. They valued her honesty. Some began to take a brotherly attitude toward her, asking her to join their activities. She was having the time of her life. After a few months, several men confided that they had crushes on her. Having learned her lesson well, Hope said no gently and said she would wait "until I'm ready to get serious."

Decision Making

Bulimarexics have great difficulty making decisions. They are outcome-oriented rather than process-oriented and terrified of making mistakes and appearing foolish. Therapy should emphasize that profiting from failure is a major concomitant of success. We all need to listen to criticism in order to grow. These women need to learn how to deal with the crashes. Therapy therefore involves help in seeing crisis as opportunity for change.

For the bulimarexic, agonizing over the outcome is part of decision making. Mary doesn't want to take that course unless she is guaranteed an A. Betty doesn't want to take up skiing unless she can race downhill after two lessons. What's missing is being able to say, "Good for me—way to go! You're working hard and getting closer to your goal—keep up the good work." When our clients confront themselves with negative messages such as "I'm afraid," we ask them to finish the sentence: "I'm afraid of . . ." Most bulimarexics have never thought this through. It hasn't dawned on them that they control their minds and don't have to act on what they feel. In life we are only judged for what we *do,* not for what we think. Recognizing this is true liberation.

To further confuse matters, even when a decision is made, bulimarexics continue to agonize. They have great difficulty standing by their decisions. Half expecting failure, they end up with self-fulfilling prophecies—their fears come true. Encouraging clients to talk about these self-defeating scripts and role-play them is an integral part of our treatment.

The Princess Syndrome

The women we treat have an extremely low tolerance for pain or emotional discomfort. Over and over they say things like: "It's unfair; why me?; I don't want any waves. I don't deserve this. I shouldn't have to deal with this." Their attempts to avoid dealing with painful situations almost always lead to bingeing. A client named Tammy called us at midnight one evening. Her car had broken down on a rural road, and she was telephoning from a restaurant nearby. She was sobbing and on the verge of bingeing. We asked her to consider what she needed *now,* thereby breaking the "poor-me syndrome." She then was able to follow through by calling the state police, a tow station, and finally a cab to pick her up. Worn out by her ordeal yet pleased with herself, Tammy was able to make the decision not to binge.

Incidentally, while it's true that mechanical problems associated with cars and machinery are a mystery to many women, the skills women failed to acquire as little girls can no longer serve as an excuse for helplessness! Such skills can be learned even more efficiently in adulthood.

The People Pleaser

At the core of bulimarexia is the need to conform. Women are taught to play to an audience—an audience that often has a cast of thousands. Self-consciousness and misinterpretation often result.

A significant number of clients, for example, refuse to engage in some physical activity they previously enjoyed if they gained a few pounds. They think all eyes are upon them at the health club as they walk through the door. The prospect of putting on a leotard or bathing suit terrifies them. Thus they withdraw at the worst possible time from the things they need most. It's helpful to point out to these women that their extreme concern is unwarranted. No doubt every woman at the health club is preoccupied with her own problems, real or perceived.

At times the people-pleasing tendencies of bulimarexics border on the ridiculous. During a recent group session, members broke into laughter after one woman realized she was also a *dog* pleaser. She had been allowing her dog to sleep on her bed (he was lonely!) even though he nightly woke her with his scratching and moving around and denied her much-needed sleep.

When women are struggling with these issues, it is helpful to ask: "Are these big people or little people in your life?" "Little people" are the less important ones or the ones for whom you lack respect. "Big people" are loved and/or respected. Thinking this through allows women to put the audience in perspective and cut down on its numbers, perhaps for the first time.

OTHER ISSUES IN THERAPY

Some of our clients have moved away from religion and their religious communities because of shame and guilt over their eating habits. We often call on pastoral counselors to help women resolve these and other spiritual issues. Frequently this leads to renewed religious interest and a new source of strength and security.

Clients may also feel the need to examine the unfinished business of the past more thoroughly. We ask them to take responsibility for this exploration and outline the areas they want to work on. Once they are coping with bingeing in the present and looking forward to the future, there is much to be gleaned from examining how past experiences have shaped present behaviors.

For example, Lorna, no longer bingeing and purging on her visits home from college, began to notice family patterns more. By refusing to participate in the same old interactions with her mother, she found they fought far less. Observing her family at dinner also provided insights. No one seemed to listen to anyone. Everyone interrupted. No one finished a conversation. Lorna began to understand how she had acquired her habit of talking loudly and quickly; feeling invisible, she was always competing for the attention of the group and rarely succeeding. Perhaps there was a clue here about problems with friends at school!

When clients reach this level of growth, they may need more time *out of therapy* to experiment with new strategies in old situations. We may begin seeing women every two weeks—and then once a month. Months may pass without a visit, but the client always knows that booster sessions are available at her request. Sometimes there is a need to work on a difficult future event—going home or interviewing for a job—sometimes a woman is experiencing rejection or failure and needs temporary support. Usually such visits are precipitated by real crises and are in themselves adaptive strategies; as therapists, we then facilitate decision making or acknowledge the good work the client has already accomplished.

THE WEEKLY GROUP EXPERIENCE

The weekly group has some advantages over the intensive workshop experience. Women can receive therapy as long as they need it, at the same time developing friendships that will sustain them outside of the therapy hour. Since most of our clients lack intimate relationships with other women, these weekly sessions help them to share their innermost fears, fantasies, and flaws with others, often for the first time.

We feel that ongoing groups should be relatively homogeneous. Now, for example, we direct a group for career women and married women, and another for high school and college students. Even with this division, there are sharp individual differences. For example, many students are in control of their home situations so that bingeing and purging are rarely problems over vacation. Others are fine during the school semester only to succumb to violent binge/purge rituals in the home atmosphere. A variety of conditions serve to initiate and maintain bingeing for different women. Individual therapy in the context of the group helps the client to recognize and understand these patterns in order to fortify herself against stress.

Our criteria for continuing groups are different from our intensive seminars. For group membership, we require some previous success in attenuating bingeing and purging. These groups are designed for "recovering" bulimarexics. It's best if women have had one-to-one therapy or intensive seminar involvement before entering a weekly group. Beginning a group with even one hopeless and helpless woman is to be avoided since pessimism and depression are contagious to all. The chronically resistant client also subtracts from the group and receives very little herself. A few years ago, we had a successful weekly group of women who had traveled some distance to attend. They were highly motivated and well-educated and had read the most up-to-date literature on eating disorders. All had been referred by professionals. We had, however, accepted one woman who could not afford individual psychotherapy. Because she was exceedingly skeptical and hostile about the progress of the others, she was a toxic influence. Ultimately, she was asked to leave the group. We finally found an appropriate referral resource, and the woman obtained individual therapy.

All this is not to suggest that we shield group members from unpleasant experiences. On the contrary, we encourage free expression of frustration and pain since such experiences often provide the most powerful incentives to change. During one of our first groups, which consisted of severe bulimarexics, one member binged *in front of* the group. The rest of the women watched in dismay. Some felt as though they were watching a videotape of themselves—and on the basis of this experience their own commitment was intensified and real progress initiated. So careful selection of candidates for therapy must take such elusive variables into account.

The First Session

All group members must agree to attend at least twelve consecutive sessions. The first session is generally quite subdued. Members assume that other women engage in similar behavior, but they have fears and fantasies about frequency, intensity, and duration of bingeing. Our first task is to outline what will be expected in the group. Honesty, respecting confidences, risk taking, and regular attendance are among the rules. We talk about what commitment means. From the first session on, we generate homework assignments involving risk taking with toxic foods, people, and situations *only when the women feel strong.* We ask them to undertake five such risks between the first and second group sessions, emphasizing the importance of "lightening up," rewarding themselves for handling difficult situations, and realizing that expectations of success may be too high.

The women are asked to meet for dinner before or after the group session. We warn them not to reach out for help this early in the game since we haven't taken up goal contracting. We ask them to take notes and use those notes, particularly during their most stressful times.

Some women are less active in the group than others; group members who hold back often make the most progress through vicarious learning. Some therapists who come to train with us have difficulty with our laissez-faire approach. They worry about the more retiring women and interpret silence as negative. In one case, Julie, a psychologist, became concerned about a group member named Mary Ann who had not said a word for two sessions. We asked Julie to express her concerns to the group. Mary Ann immediately said she was relieved that no one had tried to "put her on the hot seat." She added that she "had never worked so hard" at assimilating information and then shared several remarkable insights with the group.

We usually begin group sessions by reviewing homework assignments and often find that women with real success to report rarely fully acknowledge their accomplishments. We point out how self-defeating this is and work on more acceptable ways of reinforcing any positive action. We facilitate and examine contracting of goals with oneself or another person. By the third or fourth session, the women are eager to call on one another outside of the group. Participants may meet on Saturday mornings, for example, to jog together, thus breaking the habit of sitting at home with the temptation to binge. Once a group is settled in, we sometimes bring in new members. The veterans are eager to help the new women, show them the ropes, and demonstrate success. They become better models for new members, a mutually therapeutic situation. As established members progress, they are urged gradually to reduce attendance at sessions; however, the group is always available to them, whenever they feel the need.

COUPLE COUNSELING

These days more husbands are aware of eating disorders and are struggling with their own feelings about whether or not they can or should attempt to help the women in their lives. Increasingly, we have found it useful to offer group sessions for husbands, boyfriends, and fathers who share the women's confidence. Bill directs these groups, which have proved exceedingly helpful since some men need a forum where they can express their resentment and anger. Questions are encouraged. As with the women, individual needs are taken into account. Predictably the men's needs vary at different times; some men, for instance, may have difficulty when their women begin to change. The power relationship has been unequal. The wife, daughter, girlfriend who is bulimarexic may have acted little and pathetic (or bizarre and unpredictable), letting the man assume control. Assertiveness on the part of the woman is, therefore, not always readily accepted. Such behavior is unfamiliar and therefore suspect. Expressions of independence as well as developing relationships with other women can also be threatening.

Sometimes husbands don't feel as necessary as they did previously. In their bewilderment, some men inadvertently sabotage their mates and loved ones. Jim owned up to bringing home a bag of Twinkies after Yvonne had managed to go two weeks without bingeing or purging. Although he saw the Twinkies as a test, his real motive, as he admitted, was to "keep her from outgrowing me"—something that he had been feeling lately since Yvonne had been away from home more, busy with new activities.

A few men have difficulty accepting binge lapses once their partners are involved in therapy. These men expect "bionic" strides and need help in learning how to reinforce their partners' behaviors without expecting perfection. Special emphasis is placed upon specific goal contracts that can be agreed upon mutually so that both parties learn to tolerate mistakes and growth.

Often, it is helpful to see couples individually in order to help them learn new ways of communicating, fighting fair, and giving as well as receiving. One couple, Ted and Thelma, accomplished a great deal in only two sessions. Although Thelma had made progress in reducing the frequency of bingeing and purging, she found herself lying to Ted when she did have a lapse. Understandably, this bothered him and made him skeptical about her progress. In the contract they initiated, Thelma was to be honest with him no matter what. Ted's worry and resentment soon dissipated as Thelma consistently owned up to her lapses. Ted was able to help her, now that he knew about her difficult times. Thelma agreed to tell Ted how she wanted him to behave under various circumstances, with the stipulation that if their contract was not helpful, they would troubleshoot or abandon it. At times Thelma needed Ted to be firm; at other times a comforting hug was more appropriate. On occasion she simply needed some space. Whatever the situation, she was to tell him what she needed.

In turn, Thelma wanted to help Ted with one of his bad habits. Whenever they had a fight, Ted would bring up unfinished business. With the new contract, he agreed to try to stay in the here and now and let go of the past. Thelma also believed that Ted was too critical. He thought she was supersensitive and felt she had an inflated image of herself as an especially giving person. When was the last time she could remember telling him that she loved him or simply praising him for some accomplishment? When Ted asked this, Thelma was speechless. She had been so self-preoccupied that she failed to take enough notice of him. Many "caretaking" men, like Ted, need to lean on their partners occasionally. During the next two weeks, Thelma fulfilled her part of the contract, though Ted slipped frequently and still harped on unfinished business. However, as she changed, he began to show her more respect, and she was reinforced as a model for Ted. Ted soon mellowed, and they enjoyed a much more compatible relationship.

FAMILY THERAPY

Family therapy with bulimarexics can be very helpful, particularly when the client is living at home or is financially dependent on others. Whenever possible, visiting parents of college students should be encouraged to participate in therapy sessions. At the very least, the therapist gains awareness of family dynamics. Telephone conversations, especially before home visits or vacations, can be useful. Of course, confidentiality for the young woman must be assured.

Many parents have had bad experiences with previous therapy. One parent or both may have been discouraged from participating, not necessarily by his or her own choice, but because the therapist assumes that the father or mother is overinvolved or the client doesn't think it will help. Rapport should first be established with the client, after which parents' issues are more easily addressed. Bulimarexia is not the parents' fault. The problem lies in how the young woman perceives the parents. Most parents do not demand perfection; in fact, they would give anything to see their daughters relax and enjoy life. In our experience, few parents expect straight A's. By the same token, our clients are not generally hostile to their parents; many of these women feel close to their parents and respect them. But they need to confront and rewrite their own scripts, fraught with misplaced guilt and shame.

Some mothers want to initiate therapy for daughters. The adolescent girl is often opposed to therapy and parents don't quite know how to proceed. Should they insist that the young woman come in to see us? We ask parents what they would do if a child broke her leg and refused to be treated. They always respond: "We would put her in the car and drive her to the doctor." We ask them to respond similarly to the eating disorder. Once we have seen the girl alone, she usually becomes more amenable and receptive. If she still refuses therapy, we wait. When she is ready, she'll know where to turn. Daughters may initially agree to therapy to please the parents, but soon therapy becomes doing something for oneself.

In the first few sessions, we see the young woman alone in order to establish rapport and develop an atmosphere that's open and honest. Once this is established, we encourage the client to invite her parents to attend part of the session. With further rapport and credibility, we start to become tougher and more goal oriented. We frequently point out that it is unfair for young women to expect their parents to pay for therapy as well as for binge food. We suggest that they consider taking part-time jobs so they can pay for their own binge food. We're not asking clients to stop bingeing and purging—we are simply asking them to take more responsibility for this behavior. Often the adolescent cannot believe what she has heard. This contract in itself is often therapeutic, serving to lessen binge/purge practices whether or not the student takes a job.

So far as parents are concerned, our task here is to deter them from the sort of collusion that may have been advanced in earlier therapy. Why should the adolescent girl change if she is not in pain? Trudy's parents would not interrupt their daughter between seven and ten o'clock each evening. This was, after all, her binge/purge time. Hanna's parents spent months standing helplessly by while she consumed and then threw up more than a hundred dollars' worth of food a week. Both Trudy's and Hanna's therapists had advised the parents to leave their daughter alone because she was expressing important feelings by bingeing. Another woman, Joanna, blackmailed her parents into driving her to the supermarket after her therapy sessions. She would only agree to therapy if her parents allowed her to binge afterward. Our purpose in family therapy is to see that parents' rights are acknowledged and respected. Thus family sessions involve weekly goal contracts and being clear about the consequences of breaking the rules. Parents are encouraged to reinforce daughters' successes and to withhold rewards if the contract is broken.

SABOTAGE AND RESISTANCE

While most bulimarexics respond well to the short-term interventions we've described, others manage to sabotage themselves and resist all help. Some of these people are "professional patients"; they have been in and out of inpatient hospital programs, hypnotherapy, biofeedback, chemotherapy, and one-to-one and group treatment. Many have experienced a full range of therapeutic styles. Some have been treated with antidepressants, usually Tofranil, for periods of up to several years. The majority are still entangled in disturbed relationships and lack day-to-day survival skills.

These are women whose emotional growth has been stunted. Their mothers are often helpless and ineffectual, beset by their own psychological problems. Their fathers, who may be idolized, are likely to be distant and preoccupied. Mothers and daughters may form unhealthy symbiotic attachments. Daughters are unwilling to venture out in the world; mothers feel they cannot live without them. The majority of these women in the twenty-five to forty age group have never had an intimate relationship with a man, and social life may be nonexistent. Typically, they have a history of failures before becoming bulimarexic and have been suicidal and/or clinically depressed. Some continue to abuse drugs and/or alcohol.

Some of these women were obese as children, and the terror of being fat again is something they experience daily. They are pain phobic, professionals at avoiding the risks of daily living. Occasional forays away from the family are often unsuccessful. Time spent hiding at home serves to weaken them in all important aspects of their lives. They become even more sensitized to pain and discomfort, and so the vicious cycle continues. The behavior can be ameliorated, but family therapy will probably be necessary if only to interrupt the "enabling" cycle of the family. These women will also require long-term therapy, perhaps on an inpatient basis. The following account typifies our experience with such clients.

EMILY had been in and out of psychiatric facilities for many years before reaching out to us for help. She had been an unhappy, obese youngster and was pathologically dependent on her close-knit religious family for support. She married very young, and her misery continued. Her husband was alcoholic, physically abused her, and finally left her for another woman. Unable to cope on her own, she became seriously suicidal, and custody of her son was awarded to her husband. Her weight dropped to eighty-two pounds, and she was hospitalized for anorexia. After regaining twenty pounds, she began a five-year cycle of extreme bingeing and purging. She was hospitalized again and again, always returning to her parents' home. Many types of medication were tried as well as electroshock treatments. When we met her, she was thirty years old, living with her parents, and bingeing ten to twenty times per day.

Initially, we saw Emily three times a week for one-to-one psychotherapy but did not begin by working on her eating disorder. Instead we tried to help her monitor and change her negative thinking.

At the same time we helped her devise a structured daily schedule, with emphasis on physical exercise and ways of dealing more effectively with day-to-day problems. After Emily started to feel some sense of mastery and pleasure, we looked at her pattern of bingeing and purging. Holding off on this is important; these women need to have some successes. Working on the binge/purge cycle too soon only exacerbates their profound sense of helplessness and hopelessness. Emily, for example, first made progress in handling inactivity and boredom. She began to jog and signed up for an aerobics course. We worked out a visitation plan for her son, and she began moving closer to her child in gradual steps. After three months, Emily herself wanted to address the binge/purge cycle. We challenged her, using paradoxical techniques and saying we felt she needed to make further progress in other areas before taking this on. A few weeks later, Emily obtained a part-time job. When she *showed* this commitment, we reinforced it by agreeing to begin work on her bulimarexic behavior. With these clients, every step needs to be rehearsed and subtle sabotage maneuvers exposed.

With Emily, it was not productive to bring the family into therapy. The mother was overtly psychotic and the father seldom home. Since Emily needed to break away from this environment and develop other identities in the "real" world, we encouraged her to move into a small apartment and be on her own. She is progressing slowly but has held on to her job and sees her son regularly.

If clients are clinically depressed, we avoid working on the bulimarexia until thought distortions have been corrected and the women are more motivated and expressive. Success in saying no and setting limits paves the way for more difficult habit modification.

There is another group of women who resist making changes in their binge-eating practices. These women who rarely seem upset about anything enjoy avoidance of anxiety and settle for a relatively pain-free lifestyle. Someone is usually reinforcing their avoidance behavior. At times the woman "terrorizes" the family, which feels helpless to deal with her. These women are the most irresponsible of clients. They regularly miss appointments. They lie about their efforts and progress, often delighting in having their lies exposed. Inside these women are angry, stubborn children who hate being controlled. For years they have been the "sick" person in the family.

Joining the "Force"

When a client's progress is slow and she is not clinically depressed, paradoxical techniques can be helpful. We may tell the client that we're frustrated at the lack of progress and suggest that we have overestimated her ability to change. We may tell her that we don't want to work on bingeing and purging for a while and/or we're going to have to move a lot more slowly than we had anticipated. We may even say that we wonder whether she has what it takes to overcome her problems! Resisting again, the client's predictable reaction is anger—"I'll show them! Where do they get off saying I can't do this?" Such resistance is essential if certain clients are to be sufficiently motivated to take risks and succeed.

When a client insists that she cannot give up her "five o'clock binge," we ask her to simply delay the binge until five-thirty. If she succeeds, we suggest that she has earned the right to a super binge. If she usually eats a quart of ice cream, we ask her quite seriously to consume two quarts. In rebellion she often decides that she is not going to be controlled by the therapist. Or she may be delighted by her ability to *delay* bingeing when she was sure she couldn't and rewards herself by *not* bingeing.

A client named Jo Ellen responded to paradoxical techniques. At thirty-six, she had been bulimarexic for fifteen years and had no intention of attenuating her bingeing and purging, although she had endured a range of medical complications because of her behavior. Clients like Jo Ellen are difficult to work with. Although they make little progress, they are cheerful and energetic. Therapy is also considered chic. Tiny strides, from time to time, often serve to keep the therapy going. Jo Ellen's breakthrough came after she attended her fifteenth high school reunion, where she encountered classmates who were, as she put it, "piglike." She watched with glee as they shoveled the food into their "chubby" bodies. We pointed out that she maintained her weight dishonestly and did *no* work to achieve her size six. Imagine how it would be, we asked, if she were to return five years later to her twentieth high school reunion, having achieved a reasonable weight through hard work and honesty. Jo Ellen was astonished. She had never considered her behavior in this light, and the impact of our paradoxical injunction was dramatic. Three months later she had broken her fifteen-year cycle of daily bingeing and purging.

Most bulimarexic clients will resist or rebel at one time or another and then respond with the support and encouragement of treatment. This is to be expected since most are totally unrealistic about how change will occur. They think the therapist will wave a magic wand, and they balk once they realize that they are partners in initiating change. One client, Beth, had made almost no progress for about three weeks. Then she reported that she hadn't binged for an entire week. At our instruction, wherever she went she carried a list of twenty reasons why she did not want to binge and purge. Every time she felt like bingeing, she would pull out her list and remind herself that she did not want to binge. However, even though she had been successful that week, she felt miserable and looked terrible. It turned out that forcing herself to think constantly about not bingeing had made her feel that she would have to work like this *for the rest of her life!* If so, she decided, she wasn't interested.

People like Beth need to be reminded that new habits displace old habits gradually, often requiring months of practice but not years. Beth would have to work at staying slim, but the amount of time and energy expended would become less and less.

SUBSTANCE ABUSE AND BULIMAREXIA

One out of ten women in every group we treat has a history of alcoholism and/or drug abuse. Samantha is fairly typical. Like other women with multiple addictions, she moved from one dependent drug state to another, sometimes in the course of one day. What is remarkable is that she could function at all. In spite of her problems, Samantha was able to keep the same job for two years. Samantha would awake at 5:45 A.M. in order to get to the kitchen while it was deserted. Her parents didn't see her while she consumed every crumb she could find, and they didn't hear her when she promptly disposed of those dreaded calories in the toilet. Since she had to be at work, which is two hours away, by 8:30, she chose to bicycle there in order to burn 400 calories along the way. At 11:45, forty-five minutes before lunch, she casually picked up her tote bag and slipped into the cafeteria, where a refrigerator with a stash of brown bags provided her with her second binge of the day. When she was done, she purged.

At 4:15 P.M., fifteen minutes before the end of work, Samantha took Elavil and Stelazine prescribed for depression. She took her medication at this time so that she could stop at a bar, drink to the point of intoxication, and burn off 525 calories biking to the bar and then home. At home, since her mother had saved the leftovers, she started with them and continued with whatever else was in the refrigerator. She binged and then purged, even though her vision was now affected by her medication, and she was totally exhausted.

At 5:45 A.M., the alarm awoke her to another destructive day.

Eventually Samantha's behavior became too much for her. Severely depressed, she borrowed her parents' car and deliberately slammed it into a telephone pole at sixty miles per hour. Miraculously, she survived and soon afterward entered a drug and alcohol treatment program. The support and the consistent caring attitude and treatment provided by the staff helped her break free of both alcohol dependency and bingeing and purging. When she came to us for treatment, she had been sober for several months and except for an occasional lapse did not binge or purge. She felt she needed support more than therapy at this point and so became an enthusiastic and articulate member of a group. This participation bolstered her sense of autonomy. In time, her addictive involvements became less and less necessary and appealing.

Some clinicians believe that the prognosis is poor when bulimarexia is associated with other addictive behaviors. Others maintain that pessimism is unwarranted if the drug problem arose as an attempt to stave off bingeing or dull the pain associated with it. There are also differing views about treatment. Addiction counselors are uncertain how to treat bulimarexics who are substance abusers. Most drug and alcohol programs emphasize abstinence, but one cannot abstain totally from food. The bulimarexic has to learn—or relearn—how to eat sensibly and healthfully.

When we see multiple addictions, we insist that the substance abuse be alleviated before we will address bulimarexia. A brain that functions clearly is necessary for thinking, let alone initiating change. Once this is accomplished, the prognosis for overcoming bulimarexia has been excellent. Those who can free themselves from chemical dependency usually feel confident enough to tackle their eating disorder.

Some women become bulimarexic after gaining weight during their rehabilitation from drugs and/or alcohol. This type of weight gain, from ten to twenty pounds generally, is not at all uncommon. Others begin to abuse drugs such as cocaine to control their weight since cocaine has a profound appetite control mechanism. Still another group become substance abusers to numb the pain associated with bingeing and/or weight gain; in such cases, unexpected weight gain leads to depression—which leads to alcohol or drugs—which leads to more weight gain. Thus they avoid the depression associated with bingeing and purging and often delay or avoid overeating by taking drugs or alcohol.

People have various complex ways of remaining "unconscious" under stress. They have ways of anesthetizing themselves and denying that problems exist. The numbing reported by clients when they're bingeing is similar to the numbing provided by alcohol or drugs. Some treatment models for bulimarexia depart dramatically from our own in requiring complete cessation of the behavior. We have always believed that learning from mistakes is critical. So much of the bulimarexic's thinking is all or nothing, black or white, that relapse is inevitable and very likely to occur if treatment programs are too rigid. Indeed, that has been the case with many clients who came to us after previous treatment was unsuccessful.

TERMINATION AND RECOVERY

Throughout therapy we insist that women take notes—jot down words, phrases, and concepts that serve as building blocks to a more productive lifestyle. We point out that bulimarexic behavior has taken up much time and energy in the past that can now be devoted to *doing*—doing whatever *they* choose. Women have consistently told us how valuable their notebooks were to them after treatment. The following notes were shared with us by a former client, who, after eleven months of binge-free living, felt that her adherence to the following principles served to maintain her strides toward recovery.

Habit	Bulimarexia is *not* a disease; it is a *learned* behavior that can be unlearned.
Responsibility	Gorging and purging will continue unless the bulimarexic stops blaming other people and/or circumstances (i.e., "I flunked the exam because I binged" really means "I flunked it because I didn't study"). Take *responsibility* for the behavior.
Why	Let go of the "whys" because you can never be sure if you are right. Ask instead: "What do I get from

	gorging and purging?" Then you will have some idea of what might replace these destructive behaviors.
Past/Present/ Future	"What tense am I in?" Give up dwelling on yesterday as well as rehearsing for tragedy in the future. Devote energy and attention to the *moment.* That's where you can make an impact.
Expectations	Let go of expectations and begin *honest goal contracting.* Expectations lead to disappointment, which fosters bulimarexia. Goals do not imply outcome but represent a commitment to *trying.*
Pain	Think of pain as a precursor to *change,* not to bingeing. Learn from your pain, not how to avoid it. Don't court pain, but use it to motivate risk taking. *Acting* rather than reacting is key to the process of change.
Risk taking	Be willing to step into the unknown without being absolutely certain of the outcome. Progress is dependent upon trying new ways of living. If you don't like the outcome, you can go back to the way you were. Few things in life are irreversible.
Toxic words	Eliminate such words as *can't, forever,* and *never* from your vocabulary. They are stepping-stones to *perfectionism* and to ultimate self-defeat. There are no bionic people!
Power	Don't give up your power by allowing others to control you. Don't say yes when you really mean no. Take a careful look at your *audience.* Stop being a *people pleaser,* and start making your *own* mistakes.
Mistakes	Nobody's perfect, so when you make a mistake stay in the here and now and troubleshoot. If you don't, you're likely to make the same mistake again and again.
Sabotage	Avoid those self-destructive yet tempting states of being (i.e., isolationism, perfectionism, pessimism, and inactivity). Identify your *rackets*—those behaviors that, in the long run, feed bulimarexia.
Ask	Don't interpret! With your self-concept, you're sure to expect the worst! Learn to ask rather than to analyze.

Identity   Oneness must precede twoness! Establish your
                    identities. You are what you do. Self-respect is
                    contingent upon success experiences. Learn to
                    reinforce yourself so that growth is not based solely
                    upon interactions with others. *Be kind to yourself in
                    the face of stress* so that you can cope rather than
                    succumb to a binge. Enjoy your accomplishments.
                    Practice giving as well as accepting strokes!

These important behavioral principles are the essence of treatment. Women who truly understand them usually make a commitment to change in unique ways. However, a new beginning in
an old environment often proves difficult. Furthermore, healthy
strides need to be maintained *over time*. When they are not, it is fair
to say that therapy has been of limited value. Thus, the final aspect
of our treatment involves taking "psychological inventory." The
time has come to determine whether the well-educated client is
now capable of handling the stressful situations that she is likely to
encounter.

As a final exercise, we ask each woman to rehearse for tragedy—
that is, to live in the future. By now, each one has a list of her
salient "red lights"—the people, places, and attitudes that have invariably led to binge/purge behavior. In addition, each has delineated alternatives to bingeing. Rehearsing for the future now
represents an opportunity to apply new strategies to old situations.
The woman can prove to herself that she is a different person in an
important way.

This is a time of concerns and questions. Nearly every woman
asks us: *When (and how) will I know I am no longer bulimarexic?*
The question is natural, considering the tenacity of the
binge/purge syndrome; it represents the woman's fear that she can
never be sure she is free of the behavior. She is, of course, sub-
scribing to the belief that serious habits such as alcoholism, smok-
ing, and drug abuse must be eliminated completely if the outcome
is to be successful. However, recent research into these problems
has cast doubt on whether the all-or-nothing hypothesis is accu-

rate. As far as bulimarexia is concerned, to insist that the bulimarexic can never take one mouthful of a forbidden food is simply unwarranted, as many women will attest. So the answer to the
question of when and how bulimarexia becomes a behavior of the
past depends on the individual and the goals she sets herself. For
example, Laura, a former group member, writes: "It has been three
years since the group, and I am now cured! Oh, I still overeat on
occasion (about once a month), but I don't view it as the end of the
world, and I don't use it as an excuse to engage in the old cyclic ritual. I now like my life *most* of the time, and, although I'm still lazy
and find that I binge when I feel that way, I can deal with it because
I own that part of me. It no longer owns me!"

Jill feels: "I'm not there yet! I have cut the frequency of my
binges in half over the past year and haven't purged for over two
years, but I still feel out of control when I resort to overeating. I've
learned *a lot,* but I want more therapy, so I have negotiated a new
contract with my old therapist. We'll see how it goes."

Finally, Eve, who had been bingeing and purging for eighteen
years, had this to say thirty months after her workshop experience:
"I'll never be completely happy unless I stop this forever. I know
that this statement smacks of sabotage, and just knowing that helps
a great deal. It allows me to admit that I use eating as a way of
avoiding intimacy. I still binge once in a while (once or twice a
month), not out of habit but in order to avoid men (at the same
time, I continue to blame them for my loneliness). My purging is
far less frequent now (six times last year), and my therapy is aimed
much more at risk taking. I'm at peace with myself for the first
time in years and am grateful for that. Perhaps I will stop this
habit. However, if I don't, I can now get on with my life as I have
been doing for the last two years. I will reach out to you again if I
feel the need to stop permanently."

Thus, Laura is willing to believe that she is finished with bulimarexia, although she still overeats occasionally. She likes herself
most of the time. She has given up certain absolutes and no longer
believes that a lapse means she has failed; Laura knows that she
does not have to be perfect and indeed will never be perfect.

Jill is more tentative, not willing to call herself cured because she still binges at times. But she is motivated enough to trust a therapist to help her cut down her need to binge and is hopeful. She knows she is not there yet but has not dismissed the possibility that she can stop completely.

Eve admits to greater serenity but knows she will not be satisfied until she stops completely. However, she is not ready to make a permanent commitment. This may be quite wise since for the time being she *knows* how she is using the behavior. When she is able to be more outgoing, more of a risk taker, she will not have to fall back on bulimarexia.

The common denominator for all these women is, of course, their belief systems. Laura is confident, Jill and Eve less so. Thus despite comparable strides and strategies, these women respond to their success experiences and their failures differently.

These three women were at different stages of readiness to give up bulimarexia. Two reached out for further therapy, often a good thing. A therapist who is knowledgeable about the problem, who does not judge and measure outcome by *his or her criteria,* may be able to speed the process of change. However, therapy is not a panacea for everyone struggling with bulimarexia. Many women are not ready to work on giving up bingeing. Others are still looking for a magic solution. Still others are secretly looking for an excuse to continue, and these women seek therapy so they can claim they have tried everything. As one woman candidly put it: "I wanted to be able to say, 'Well, I worked with the experts, but I'm still bingeing.' " These women are, of course, covertly relying upon someone else to make everything right instead of tackling the problem themselves.

Fortunately, the majority of bulimarexic women are intelligent. When therapy directly exposes their sabotage maneuvers, most will—at some time—try alternatives to bingeing *on their own.* Women we have interviewed only once have called months later to tell us that they have been binge-free since they chose to initiate the call. The mere act of picking up the phone and calling us appeared to give them the strength they needed to begin the change. In effect, that phone call represented the first risk.

Recently, we have begun "booster treatment" programs with former clients to work on specific issues and unfinished business of the sort expressed by Jill and Eve. So far this format has proved to be an effective adjunct to our workshops. The rewards are significant for us also since these programs enable us to keep in touch with many women we have come to know and respect. The following letter, addressed to the other members of a particular workshop, is illustrative:

Dear Friends:

I am writing to you to share some of my feelings and experiences since our workshop and to tell you that I am celebrating over five years of freedom from bulimarexia! There have been some very tense, anxious moments, but I've gotten through them without resorting to my former way of coping with a good ole "binge and purge" session. I am writing to say I care, and I hope that I can somehow send you some energy or strength, if you need it, to overcome this habit that we have lived with so long.

I have decided to work with other women who, like us, are trying hard to free themselves of the behavior that we found so consuming. In talking with many women, I find I am most often asked what I have now replaced the behavior with. I wish I could say that another behavior fits the slot perfectly and relieves the inner tension as well. It simply isn't that easy. I think more than anything I have replaced bingeing and purging with freedom, direction, and health. I look back on my seven years of bulimarexia as a sentence in which I was ruled, controlled, dominated, driven, and obsessed by a behavior that did not allow me to get on with my life, to accept responsibility for it, and, quite frankly, to grow up! That is my freedom from the behavior, and I see my life moving in a direction in which I am leading and not being led as before.

I have gotten through these past two years by taking them a day at a time. (There were some particularly difficult moments in which I focused on an hour at a time!) I have learned how to reach out when I feel weak and to allow others to help me by telling them what I need. I have called my husband and my sister when I was anxious or scared that bingeing might reemerge and asked them for a shot of energy and strength to get back my resolve. I have kept myself from giving in to the moment and blaming it on all those external forces. I have actually walked out of my house leaving behind the kitchen and other "trigger places" to take a walk or a ride from the stimulus of set-up situations.

Occasionally, I look back with sadness at having lost seven years of really productive living. Years when my priorities and focus were so out of line! I am ashamed of the abuse I put my body through, but I applaud my success! I have learned that it's nice to get strokes from others, but learning to stroke yourself is as important and as gratifying. I can still recreate the warmth of our weekend together in which we shared our strengths and weaknesses, where we learned that being helpless and weak had only fed our habits and made us dependent and victimized by our own design.

I am still very concerned with being thin, but I am working hard on not putting all my energy into bodily perfection. I am trying to relax more, which is very hard for me, but a real goal yet to reach.

I close with the hope that this letter finds you stronger and more determined in your efforts to be free of bulimarexia. I hope I have shared enough of myself to give you a sense of the happiness I have now found and the tremendous satisfaction that I feel at having beaten this habit. I would love to hear from you. I care, I'm with you, and I'm hoping that you are celebrating too!

How Loved Ones Can Help

Other questions college students frequently ask are: *How will I deal with my parents and my friends when I return home? How will I handle it when they ask, "What have you learned from therapy?"* It is natural for concerned loved ones to ask this question bluntly and directly. And it is natural for the bulimarexic woman, who hopes she will abandon the behavior entirely, to attempt to answer as directly and completely as possible. But though immediately asking the woman what she has learned may be legitimate, it can also be premature. How is the bulimarexic to know what she has learned until she has had a chance to apply her new knowledge and accumulate some successes? If she says, "I know I can quit," her expectations are probably unrealistic, at least at this time. One mistake and she is doomed. It would be much better if she answered in a more measured, provisional, and realistic way. Consider how nineteen-year-old Betsy answered the loaded question "What have you learned?" Her letter to us describes what she said to her parents:

Well folks, I'm not sure. I have learned a lot about a part of me that I don't like anymore, but I also think I have consistently underestimated that part. I now think that I will need some help if I am to permanently overcome bulimarexia. I must do most of the work myself because I have chosen to binge. Drs. White will continue to support me and so will some of the women from the group, and I think I know how you can best help me. I may make some mistakes; so might you. If so, I want to learn from them so I don't keep making the same ones over and over again.

I have not binged since I left treatment, and I feel strange physically. I want an appointment with our doctor. I want to be honest about the *whole thing* because I may have harmed myself by all of this. I also want to get back into my life as you have been urging me to. But, Daddy, I don't like jogging, I just like the talks we have when we run. I don't want to give them up but I do want to get back into swimming and I wish you and Mom would join me. I am not happy with my summer job, so I'm going to look for another. I have no expectations but I want to use my savings to pay for graduate school in order to motivate me to begin living again.

I don't want to move out as I planned. I need your support. I need you to trust me again despite past deceit and disrespect. I intend to try to be honest because unless I do, I'll slow myself down for sure. I would like to try these things for six months and then see how I'm doing. Will you help me?

Betsy's parents were willing to help but skeptical. As it turned out, she was not binge-free during her summer vacation. However, she troubleshot her mistakes and with the help of her parents is now a graduate student and has been binge-free for a year. Her life is filled with activities she enjoys, and she says: "I just don't have the time or the paralyzing inclination anymore!"

Betsy's clear statement about her immediate needs and goals

was refreshing. She included rather than excluded her parents in her plans, with the result that they felt less anger and resentment toward her. Betsy's father wrote to us: "We are so pleased to have our daughter back. She left as an angry, frightened, unapproachable child and returned as a woman to be respected! We have played a small part in that metamorphosis and, as a result, feel like a family for the first time!"

Betsy's commitment represents an active pursuit of a better lifestyle rather than a passive plea for attention. We were delighted but not surprised by the outcome.

We are often asked what parents, husbands, friends, and lovers can do to help the bulimarexic recover. By now it should be clear that very little of value can be done to or for the bulimarexic. Advice, recommendations, and threats only cause the woman to be more defiant of or dependent on those who are trying to help. Well-intentioned loved ones often set themselves up for a great deal of pain and frustration when they assume the role of caretaker. An exceptionally bright and competent attorney, the mother of one of our clients, decided that she was partially to blame for her daughter's behavior and became a "social policeman" by installing locks on kitchen cabinets for three weeks in order to "make it easier for Naomi to control herself." In so doing, the mother removed the temptation (food) and also monitored her daughter most evenings (with intermittent help from her silently begrudging husband). Naomi engaged in a variety of bizarre behaviors during this time but did not binge. The mother felt sure that her daughter was at long last in control. Sanctions were lifted, and that same day Naomi engaged in her worst binge ever. The mother, shocked and disillusioned, sought professional help and was advised to hospitalize Naomi immediately. After two months in the psychiatric ward of a major metropolitan hospital, Naomi emerged angry, resentful, and feeling more hopeless than ever. Bingeing and purging intensified. Family rapport was seriously jeopardized despite the fact that these three people had been fairly close one year earlier.

The bottom line for those who know or care about a bulimarexic is this: Do not take responsibility for her behavior by trying to fix her! If you fail, you and she will both feel you are incompetent. If you succeed, the "victim" will be dependent upon you. It is a no-win situation that is exceedingly difficult to resist, particularly for well-integrated, successful, caring people. The bulimarexic must initiate the process of change by herself, making a commitment to doing something on her own behalf.

WEIGHT GOALS AND NUTRITION

When women ask, "How much should I weigh?" we tell them that the female body requires a certain fat level to support its reproductive functions and maintain the necessary hormones. Bulimarexics may need to settle for a weight that is higher than they would wish because the body's metabolism shifts according to the body's needs. In other words, the body can fight weight loss and gain.

In addition, certain body "flaws" characteristic of an individual may persist despite dieting, spot exercising, and massage. A pear-shaped woman, for instance, who loses twenty pounds may still have a pear-shaped configuration. Perhaps with the help of therapy, women will become less rigid in their assumptions about what is acceptable or unacceptable as far as body image is concerned. They need to learn that they are more than just their body size. Heart, spirit, and mind count, and women must start acting as though they believe this.

Some of our colleagues say that bulimarexics need to establish a weight goal about 10 percent below their highest weight before the onset of the eating disorder. Instead of focusing on a specific weight, we suggest a weight *range,* one that does not require chronic dieting to maintain. Recovery from bulimarexia seems to be linked to compromise and flexibility in this area.

What should I eat and how should I eat are other questions we are often asked. Most bulimarexics starve themselves in the daytime (and then binge at night)—a pattern that makes no physiological sense. During starvation periods, body metabolism slows down to conserve energy. When this occurs, less energy is required. Throughout the day, the body needs energy, not only for movement but also for the basic bodily functions such as heartbeat, brain activity, respiration, and muscular and nervous coordination. Calories are more efficiently burned during periods of activity rather than in the evening when most people are least active. Therefore, it makes more sense to have the energy derived from food available when the body is most active rather than depriving it when it needs this energy.

Skipping breakfast and/or lunch causes listlessness, apathy, and decreased concentration. When the body is starved, fat stores and protein are broken down for energy. Although these stores can be called upon, when necessary, they are no substitute for the dietary carbohydrates needed for certain body functions. For instance, brain cells and cells of the eye lens and nerve tissue depend specifically on glucose as a main source of energy. Under certain conditions, an extremely low blood glucose level may affect the brain, and drowsiness, fatigue, coma, and death may occur.

When little or no carbohydrates are consumed, the body adapts by deriving energy from the tissues and fat. When excess amounts of protein are used for energy, toxic levels of the waste product urea build up, and this excess urea must then be removed by the kidneys. In addition, ketone bodies (chemical byproducts) produced from the metabolism of fats (fatty acid oxidation) lead to ketosis, a metabolic acidosis, which leads to an increased production of ammonia by the kidneys and a greater loss of nitrogen by the body (Shils and Young 1988). Thus the kidneys become overworked. At the same time, an adequate amount of protein is not available for tissue repair.

To ensure a healthy recovery and long-lasting good eating habits, it is important to get the right balance of macronutrients (carbohydrates, proteins, and fats) in the diet. Recommendations for these nutrients include 50 to 55 percent of calories coming from carbohydrates, approximately 20 percent of calories from protein, and 20 to 30 percent of calories from fat. Carbohydrate sources should be high in fiber and include fresh fruits and vegetables, whole grain breads and cereals, pasta, rice, potatoes, and legumes (beans and peas). Low-fat milk and yogurt are sources of both carbohydrates and proteins. Other protein choices include lean meats and cheeses, eggs, peanut butter, and tofu. Vegetarians need to ensure that their protein intake is adequate and that they get complete proteins throughout a twenty-four-hour period.

Of the three macronutrients, fat is the most difficult to reintroduce into the diet of eating-disordered clients since food is viewed as "fattening," and fat is considered "bad." Some fats, however, are good and indeed essential for life. Dietary fats contribute fat-soluble vitamins like A,D,E, and K, essential fatty acids, phospholipids, and sterols, which are necessary for function of all tissues. Lack of dietary fats contributes to loss of body fat and a decreased production of estrogen in women, which can eventually lead to osteoporosis and disturbances in the reproductive cycle. Good fats include monounsaturated and polyunsaturated fats, found primarily in vegetable oils, nuts and seeds, and avocados. Research suggests that monounsaturated fats (such as canola, olive, and peanut oils) have protective mechanisms against heart disease. Bad fats are the saturated fats found primarily in fatty meats, whole-milk products (including cheese, butter, sour cream, and cream cheese), tropical oils (palm and coconut), and foods made with hydrogenated vegetable oils. Current recommendations by the American Heart Association are to keep saturated fat intake at less than 10 percent of the total fat per day.

A well-balanced diet also includes an adequate amount of vitamins and minerals. Iron, calcium, and zinc are of particular concern since they are all vital for proper growth and maturation in adolescents and young adults. Iron is needed for the production of red blood cells, and iron stores can be depleted easily during menses. Recommended daily iron allowances are 15 mg per day; food sources include meats and fortified cereals. Calcium is essential to the development of strong bones and teeth; new recommendations are approximately 1,200 mg per day for the adolescent and young adult. Dairy products, especially milk and yogurt, are excellent sources of calcium, but it can also be found in salmon (with bones), sardines, tofu, broccoli, and many calcium-fortified foods. Zinc, which is essential for many metabolic pathways, is found in meats, eggs, liver, and seafood and to a lesser extent in whole grains. Recommendations for zinc are 12 mg per day.

Although they are not a substitution for good food choices, a multivitamin-mineral supplement may help in the initial stages of refeeding to ensure that nutrient needs are met.

Here are some tips for a rational approach to eating, based on balance, moderation, and flexibility:

1. Stay away from fad diets. Control is best achieved by changing eating habits and maintaining the new habits.
2. Don't deprive your body of necessary calories. The body needs approximately fifteen calories per pound of body weight for a person engaging in moderate daily activity—e.g., walking or a half hour of aerobic dancing.
3. Expect to have strong emotional reactions when you attempt to lessen or stop your binge/purge behavior. Bingeing has a deadening anesthetizing impact, and feelings will begin to emerge once the binge/purge cycle is attenuated.
4. Do not diet when you make the decision to stop bingeing and purging. Dieting will only cause feelings of deprivation and lead to a binge. Instead, concentrate on normalizing eating behaviors. Restrain yourself from weighing in daily. Once a week should be enough.
5. Eat three meals a day, and incorporate two small snacks in your eating plan if desired. Do not ever starve yourself. Distribute calories evenly throughout the day by increasing the frequency of meals.
6. Eat a variety of foods, and eat them at specific times. Don't eliminate carbohydrates because they provide the most readily available source of glucose. Reduce intake of simple carbohydrates and increase your intake of complex carbohydrates. Sugars—the simple carbohydrates—and complex carbohy-

drates, which include starches, have approximately the same caloric content. However, most foods high in sugar content—like candies and many desserts—lack other nutrients such as vitamins and minerals. The foods that are high in complex carbohydrates—breads, cereals, dry beans, peas, potatoes—contain these essential nutrients.

7. Reduce the amount of salt in your diet. Sodium acts like a sponge and pulls excess fluid into the blood vessels, causing the heart to pump harder. In addition, fluid may be forced outside the blood vessels, causing edema (swelling) of the hands, feet, and legs. Weight gain due to excess fluid causes anxiety for those carefully monitoring their weight and may also lead to an increase in blood pressure and further problems.

   Substitutes for salt: Mrs. Dash seasoning mixes, pepper, lemon juice, onion, garlic, vinegar, parsley, and other herbs and spices.

8. Increase your intake of fiber. Adding fiber to your diet can be accomplished simply by consuming more fresh fruits (especially those with skins), raw vegetables, and whole grain bread and cereal products. A fiber-rich, nutritious, low-calorie snack is hot-air popped popcorn.

9. The cheapest and most natural beverage is water. Diet drinks are safe in moderate amounts, twelve to twenty-four ounces daily, but an overconsumption puts added strain on the bladder. Some diet sodas are high in sodium, caffeine, and phosphorus (which can compete with calcium and result in calcium loss from the bones), so moderate use is advised. Alcoholic beverages are high in calories and deficient in nutrients, so intake of these should be limited to one or two standard-sized drinks daily. It is recommended that everyone drink sixty-four fluid ounces (eight glasses) of water per day.

10. Consume the number of calories necessary for proper bodily functions. Restricting calories to fewer than 1,200 per day just slows down the metabolic process because the body begins conserving energy; therefore, weight gain will occur when calories are increased to a normal level. Instead of restricting

your intake, it is better to increase your amount of physical exercise.

11. Plan a number of interesting activities (besides eating) for those times when you may be bored or restless.

12. Be realistic about the body structure you were born with. Some people just have larger bones than others, and no amount of dieting will ever change that. Work on developing self-confidence.

13. Keep trigger foods in opaque containers or simply out of the house until you feel more in control of your eating patterns.

14. Incorporate trigger foods into your diet gradually. Eat small servings of the foods you were accustomed to bingeing on.

15. When possible, eat with other people and do not engage in other activities such as watching television or reading while eating. Enjoy the social aspect of eating. Make eating a pleasurable experience—notice the colors, the smells, and the flavors of foods, and savor each bite.

16. As you feel more confident about managing food, experiment with eating out. Try to shake the thoughts that food is bad, that diet is a four-letter word. Remember: Food is fuel, food is medicine. Concentrate on the benefits of a healthy diet and an improved quality of life!

17. A normal amount of exercise such as aerobic dancing three times weekly is more beneficial in long-term weight control than a strict diet regimen.

Clients often ask us to recommend an exercise program. We usually recommend aerobic classes and/or weight-training programs like Nautilus. Both require *days off* from exercise in order to rest the body and allow muscles to recover and grow. According to Dr. Ellington Darden, director of research for Nautilus Sports, athletes need at least forty-eight but no more than ninety-six hours of rest between training sessions, and workouts should be strenuous but no longer than twenty to thirty minutes. Thus working out three days a week and resting on the other days is an excellent routine. Too much exercise is counterproductive and results in a much slower growth of muscles. For our clients—many of whom are compulsive exercisers—the emphasis on rest and recovery is exceptionally therapeutic.

One great advantage to muscle conditioning is that it increases the muscles' ability to burn fat as fuel. As the body demands more energy, fat metabolism increases. People who have well-developed muscles and are in good shape find it easier to keep off excess fat.

A muscle-building program allows bulimarexic women to adjust to a higher weight than their "ideal." Because muscle weighs more than fat, women are encouraged to use the mirror in a positive way rather than relying on the bathroom scale to determine how they should feel about themselves. For the borderline anorexic/bulimic client, muscle building provides a reassuring way to accept a higher weight goal.

QUESTIONS ABOUT FOOD

Here is a list of questions that clients with eating disorders frequently ask nutritionists:

Q. How many calories do I need per day for normal functioning and/or how many calories do I need per day to prevent weight gain?

A. Calorie needs are based on a person's age, activity level, and nutrient needs. Because adolescents are in an active state of growth, their calorie needs are much higher than those of people in their early twenties and thirties. Recommended nutrient intakes for an adolescent female between the ages of fourteen to eighteen ranges from 1,500 to 3,000 calories with a median intake of 2,200 per day. The more active an individual is, the greater her calorie needs are. Weight gain during adolescence, especially between the ages of thirteen and fifteen, is essential. As growth slows, calorie needs diminish and weight begins to stabilize. At this stage, calorie needs can be estimated based on the formula: 15 calories per pound of body weight for maintenance, with an increase of 20 calories per pound for a moderately active person. Calorie intake should never be less than 1,200 calories per day regardless of body weight or activity level. If weight loss is desired, then calorie requirements are decreased by 500 calories per day to allow a one pound loss per week, and conversely calorie requirements are increased by 500 per day to allow for a weekly weight gain of one pound.

Q. What is considered a healthy weight gain or weight loss on a weekly or monthly basis?

A. A slow, long-lasting weight gain or weight loss is most desirable and should consist of no more than one half to one pound per week or two to four pounds per month.

Q. Do I have to eat beef—or any meat, for that matter—to be healthy?

A. Beef—like pork, chicken, and turkey—is a good source of protein. And protein is an essential nutrient responsible for hundreds of processes in the body, including the growth and maintenance of muscles and other tissues and proper function of the immune system. Although we can make some proteins on our own, many cannot be made without essential amino acids—protein building blocks—provided by our diet. These essential amino acids can be found in both animal and vegetable foods; however, the catch is that *all* of the essential amino acids can be eaten in a three-ounce serving of lean meat, while a vegetable serving may only have half of the essential amino acids needed. Meat, therefore, is considered a complete protein. Vegetable sources can become complete proteins by protein complementation: combining two foods to make a complete protein. The classic example of protein complementation is red beans and rice. In addition, many vegetarians include eggs, milk, and cheese in their diets, all of which provide a complete protein source. A vegetarian diet can be an excellent source of protein, and its health benefits make it a desirable option to eating meat, as long as one is well-informed on which foods combine to produce complete proteins.

Q. How many grams of fat do I need each day? What are good fats and bad fats?

A. Fat gram determination is based on the amount of calories eaten per day—generally fat needs are 20 to 30 percent of the total calories. For example, a 1,200 calorie diet would consist of 27 to 40 grams of fat per day, while an 1,800 calorie diet would consist of 40 to 60 grams of fat per day. Like proteins, there are certain fats (essential fatty acids) that cannot be produced by our bodies and must be obtained from foods. What counts is to emphasize monounsaturated and polyunsaturated fats and avoid saturated fats.

Q. How many calories do you have to use to burn a gram of fat?

A. You must expend nine calories to "burn up" one gram of fat.

Q. What is the best diet to follow for a recovering bulimic/anorexic?

A. Generally, I encourage a well-balanced diet with frequent feedings throughout the day. Daily intake includes five to seven servings of whole grains, three to five servings of fresh fruits and vegetables, two to three servings of low-fat dairy products, two servings of a three-ounce lean meat or meat alternative, 2 to 3 servings of a mono- or polyunsaturated fat (for example, butter or oil) and 1/2 to 1 serving of nuts, seeds, and legumes. In some cases, nutritional supplement may be necessary to initiate weight gain in the anorexic who is as much as 15 percent below her usual body weight. Each meal should include choices from two or more food groups. Frequent feedings (three meals with two to three snacks) allow for an even distribution of calories throughout the day to help fuel the body during times of increased energy needs. This helps to maintain—and at times boost—the body's metabolism. It prevents the fatigue, light-headedness, and lack of concentration associated with long periods of fasting or with lumping all the calories in one meal. Frequent feedings tend to prevent feelings of deprivation and hunger that can trigger a binge. Because meals are smaller, refeeding is not as overwhelming for the anorexic, who is used to eating little or nothing all day.

Q. How should foods be prepared?

A. The less a food is processed, the better. For example, a whole peach has greater nutritional value than canned peaches in heavy syrup. The process of heating the fruit during canning destroys the cell wall, allowing for a loss of fiber and vitamins. The heavy syrup contains nothing more than simple sugar that contributes only empty calories. Another example is choosing a baked or boiled potato over instant mashed potatoes. Again, more nutrients and fiber are present in the unprocessed baked potato. Avoid fried foods and foods smothered in white or cheese sauces. Vegetables are best eaten raw or lightly steamed. Meats should be baked, broiled, or grilled. When sautéing foods, use a good vegetable oil rather than butter or a stick margarine.

Q. Is it OK to sometimes have a "bad" food?

A. There is room in any sensible diet for an occasional dessert, an order of french fries, or a plate of fettucini Alfredo as long as each food is eaten in moderation and does not trigger feelings of guilt or lead to a binge. Like "good" foods, these foods can be enjoyed and savored.

Q. Why do I eat more of a food if it is low fat or fat free?

A. We often assume that as long as a food has little or no fat, we can eat it as much as we want, since we regard fat in foods is the primary culprit for weight gain and obesity. This is an assumption that we must dispel because these foods still contribute calories to our diet, and too many calories are generally the reason we gain weight.

Q. If I am starving myself, will vitamins and other supplements keep me healthy enough? If I take calcium supplements, will I still need to drink milk?

A. Vitamin and mineral supplementation will not keep an anorexic healthy enough if she is starving herself. Vitamins and minerals are simply micronutrients—nutrients that we need in small amounts to prevent nutritional deficiencies. They cannot provide the carbohydrates, proteins, and fats we need to survive on a daily basis. In addition, nutrients present in supplements are not as readily digested and absorbed as nutrients in their natural state—that is, in foods. Calcium present in supplements provides a certain percent of elemental calcium, but it is not as beneficial as the calcium we get from a glass of skim milk or from eight ounces of yogurt, nor can it provide the carbohydrates and proteins we get from these foods. (And of course supplements cannot compare to savoring a cold glass of milk after a peanut butter sandwich or a bowl of tangy yogurt topped with fresh fruit.)

Q. If I haven't eaten in a while and then eat, why do I get constipated?

A. This problem is an example of the old adage "If you don't use it, you lose it." Our digestive tract is composed of many different muscles that move food from the mouth, down to the stomach, to the small intestines, and eventually to the colon and rectum as waste. When we don't eat, these muscles lose their ability to move food efficiently. Constipation can also result from a low fiber diet and/or lack of adequate water consumption. To prevent constipation, slowly introduce fiber into your diet until you reach 25 to 30 grams per day, and drink at least eight glasses of water per day.

9.

Anorexia Nervosa:
Sociocultural Perspectives

Women have always been conditioned to take a personal responsibility for problems in their lives whose roots are social. After devoting my practice to treating eating-disordered clients over a span of twenty-five years (as well as specializing in other women's issues), I believe powerful socialization rituals force women to internalize confusing demands. It is this brainwashing/training beginning in childhood that creates a vulnerability to depression, inadequate coping strategies, excessive worrying, and "thinking disorders"—low self-esteem, self-hatred/body hatred, and the feeling that whatever is achieved is *still not good enough.*

The problem with the literature on eating disorders is that it perpetuates hopelessness and helplessness in its emphasis on disease and individual and familial deficits. Eating-disordered women and their families who read this literature are set up for failure and a self-fulfilling prophecy. Rather than individual psychopathology, I see discouraged girls who are in enormous pain. They are no different from other depressed teenagers (without eating disorders), self-mutilators, and teenagers who keep their problems to themselves.

Anorexia and bulimia are two very distinct problems with many commonalities that play out on a continuum or spectrum of eating disorders. Both have similar biological, psychological, and cultural components. The most obvious cultural mandate fueling eating disorders is the expectation that women achieve an ideal weight that over the years has become thinner and *is virtually im-*

possible to maintain. For almost thirty years women have dutifully attempted to satisfy society's demands. Those women who do must experience an absolute obsessional vigilance over their diet and body. Advertising, movies, magazines, and many television programs feature emaciated women, whom *Glamour* magazine labeled "The Superstarves," as models. A young girl's struggle to emulate them is more likely to lead to an eating disorder than to the social success and fulfillment she yearns for.

THE APPALLING STATISTICS

Ninety-five percent of individuals with eating disorders are female. The increasing incidence is seen most dramatically in young white females from upper social classes. Black women comprise approximately 3 percent, the majority of whom are from professional families. Other sociocultural and ethnic groups will no doubt be more evenly represented in the future if body shape and attitudes about body weight do not undergo a significant transformation. The American Anorexia and Bulimia Association estimates that every year one million women develop eating disorders, and 150,000 die of anorexia. It has the highest death rate for any psychiatric disorder—perhaps 5 to 15 percent die during treatment.

Now researchers are also pointing out a cumulative impact that may cause the death rate to be as high as 20 percent. Women may appear to survive anorexia only to succumb to an early death years later—the end result of intense abuse of their bodies, especially the heart. In a study published in *Acta Psychiatric Scandinavia,* Swedish researcher S. Theander found anorexic patients had a lifetime mortality of approximately 20 percent above that of a control population. Anorexia affects 5 to 10 percent of all American women, with six times that number of college students suffering from bulimarexia. Several studies estimate at least 20 percent of American college women may binge and purge on a regular basis. The age of peak onset is typically fourteen to seventeen years of age.

In the United Kingdom the story is similarly grim. According to Naomi Wolf, there are 3.5 million females with eating disorders, with six to eight thousand new cases reported each year. In many professions, anorexia and bulimarexia are typical behaviors. Dancers, models, and many actresses are especially prone to these disorders. Joan Ryan, author of *Little Girls in Pretty Boxes* (1996), reports that eating disorders are rampant in girls who participate in gymnastics and ice skating, while male athletes are largely unaffected.

Body dissatisfaction, a precursor to eating disorders, has become the norm in females. By age thirteen, 53 percent of girls are unhappy with their bodies and feel they are "too fat." By age eighteen the percentage has jumped to an astonishing 78 percent who are dissatisfied with their bodies.

Ten years ago eating disorders rarely affected women under the age of fifteen. Today they are fast becoming a normative epidemic in girls aged seven through twelve. A 1995 nutrition monitoring report found young girls in this age group are evidencing severe malnutrition and are obsessed with their size, shape, and weight. In the late 1980s studies discovered 80 percent of fourth grade girls in the San Francisco area were "watching their weight," with many also dieting. Another study of three thousand adolescents found two-thirds of the girls aged thirteen to eighteen were trying to lose weight. A study published in the March 1999 issue of the journal *Pediatrics* found two-thirds of girls in grades five through twelve said magazine photos influence their notion of the ideal figure. Of the 548 girls only 29 percent were actually considered overweight, but 66 percent wanted to lose weight. Those who consistently read these fashion magazines were three times more likely to exercise and lose weight than infrequent readers and three times more likely to have unrealistic body expectations (reported in the *Roanoke Times,* March 2, 1999).

Thus ten years later the moral imperative of starvation and the tyranny of the ideal image are even more compelling, leading to the deaths of younger and younger female children. What if it were young men instead? In *The Beauty Myth* (1991), Naomi Wolf raises the specter of a male epidemic of eating disorders: Thousands of

men are dying; how would America react to its sons of privilege—
our future—committing suicide in this manner? She predicts there
would be an "emergency" response—congressional hearings, the
best experts money could hire. She contrasts this with the young
anorexic women today dying from "institutional catatonia."

The Challenge of Anorexia

For many years I resisted treating anorexics. These girls frightened
me, and I was frightened for them. Working with them was grueling, unrelenting, and often frustrating. It was almost impossible
to leave work at work. I would find myself worrying obsessively
about one client or another, fearful that they were going to die
and/or I would be sued for malpractice. These were clients who did
not want to be there, in your office, working with you, and they
utilized enormous denial and resistance equal to that of alcoholics.
It was often difficult to form a therapeutic alliance, and rarely did
I receive any type of "strokes," or reinforcements, as I did with
other clients. They often lied to me or cheated—one client put
pennies in her panties, another wore a weight belt, and many tried
drinking copious amounts of water prior to sessions to "make
weight." Every time I started thinking I knew all of the tricks of the
trade, I would find out I had been deceived.

I certainly was not alone. There have been studies indicating
that clinicians who treat patients with anorexia nervosa frequently
feel helpless, frustrated, and stressed. This is especially true when
clients continue to lose weight in spite of the therapist's best efforts.
When residents at Massachusetts General Hospital in their first
year of training of medicine, psychiatry, and pediatrics were asked
to rate their emotional reaction to clients with diabetes, obesity,
and anorexia, they were much more negative about anorexics than
the other populations (Brotman, Stern, Herzog 1984). Cohler
(1977) has suggested psychotherapy with anorexic clients may
elicit the most intense emotional reactions encountered in a therapeutic relationship. Maria Selvini Palazzoli, one of the first Euro-
pean physicians to write about anorexia nervosa, observed that

aggressive feelings in therapists may become expressed in the form of "therapeutic pessimism" and even punitive retaliation (1978).

For years Bill's and my intensive workshops with bulimarexics kept me too busy to deal with the more difficult problems of anorexia. In the late 1980s and early 1990s, however, as managed care began to erode inpatient eating-disorder programs, I found myself not having any referral resources available for anorexics. Also, there were so many variations on the theme of an eating disorder that it was no longer possible to neatly separate bulimarexics from anorexics. Fully 50 percent of anorexics have episodes of binge eating, while bulimarexics purge via long periods of starvation and/or excessive exercise, and as many as 50 percent of bulimarexics may have a history suggestive of anorexia. I began to gather my resources together in order to develop a team approach to the treatment of anorexia. I turned to Dr. William Ball, who had been my primary medical consultant with bulimarexics for years, for ongoing medical management and evaluation of anorexic clients. Pat Young, a nutritional consultant, became a critical part of this treatment team, along with Dr. Neil Dubner, who prescribed medications for my clients when it was necessary.

As time went on, I developed more confidence in my ability to treat anorexics on an outpatient basis, and my optimism was enhanced considerably by a television program in 1994 on *20/20* about Peggy Claude-Pierre and her treatment program for anorexics at the Montreux Counselling Centre in British Columbia, Canada. I was mesmerized and horrified at the same time as I watched this attractive mother of two daughters—both of whom almost died of anorexia—lift, carry, and gently caress sixty-five-pound, barely alive skeletons, gushing words of love and affection, rocking them to sleep, feeding them. These were girls who had been given up on, girls whose families were experiencing unimaginable anguish and horror.

Ms. Claude-Pierre had started the center in 1988 after becoming completely disillusioned by the attitude and interpretations of professionals who attempted to treat her own daughters. They ran the gamut from concluding that her daughters were manipulative, selfish, and attention-seeking to telling her no cure was possible. She researched the literature and found that none of the issues or explanations about etiology made any sense. She was turned off by the punishing, coercive behavior-modification programs, forced eating, and reliance on drugs. Finally Ms. Claude-Pierre decided to tackle the negative mindset of her daughters, which she called "confirmed negativity condition" through intense, around-the-clock cognitive restructuring, "reinforcing that small kernel of hope I knew was there." After successfully treating her daughters, who completely recovered, Ms. Claude-Pierre expanded the clinic to provide a "localized environment of unconditional support." She devised a medically monitored, one-on-one, twenty-four-hours-a-day individualized care plan for these acutely ill patients. The *20/20* program was not only heartrending but also enormously uplifting and optimistic, showing me that treatment-resistant anorexics—the sickest and most chronic clients of all—could make a complete recovery.

How is Ms. Claude-Pierre's program able to succeed where all others have failed these clients? Its success seems tied to constant *reverse brainwashing* in the form of cognitive therapy; enormous love, respect, affection, and unconditional regard; nutritional rehabilitation; and a year or more of follow-up psychotherapy, support, education, and resocialization experiences.

WHAT CAUSES ANOREXIA NERVOSA?

When I began to research the literature on anorexia I found it enormously depressing, pessimistic, and often condescending in its description of anorexics as "immature, manipulative, obsessional in character, attention seeking, rigid, and developmentally arrested."

Developmental Deficits and Traumatic Loss

Overwhelmingly, contemporary eating-disorder clinicians view anorexia as a disorder of adolescent development based on the inability to cope with the demands of that period, particularly the need to develop a clearly defined personal identity and sense of personal competence. The family is seen as fostering an extraordinary emphasis on achievement and external appearance. Underneath this "false self" anorexics are described as feeling weak, unworthy, and obligated to live up to what they perceive as being relentless demands for perfection. These researchers acknowledge that anorexia nervosa begins with a diet, which at the start is indistinguishable from efforts by thousands of other adolescents to lose weight. However, because of the anorexic's "developmental deficits," dieting provides a false sense of mastery and control. And because the refusal of food causes conflicts and confrontations within the family, the anorexic is also seen as powerfully manipulative and deriving secondary satisfaction from these symptoms. It seems to me these views are not the whole story.

Hilda Bruch was one of the earliest clinicians to formulate the developmental-deficit theory about anorexia. Psychiatrically, she viewed the condition closer to narcissism or schizophrenia than neurosis. She also blamed feminism for creating impossible demands and role confusion that led to dieting and anorexia nervosa. She wrote: "Girls whose early upbringing has prepared them to become clinging-vine wives suddenly are expected at adolescence to prove themselves as women of achievement. This seems to create severe personal self-doubt and basic insecurity. In their submissive way they 'choose' the fashionable dictum to be slim as a way of proving themselves as deserving" (1985). Contemporary clinicians like Steven Levenkron (1982) present anorexia nervosa as an obsessional disorder, while family systems models blame dysfunctional interactions among family members as predisposing. Much of the early research on personality characteristics and paternal and familial dynamics was characterized by poor methodology; recent research, by Garfinkle et al. (1993) has found that parents of young anorexic clients differ little from normal controls.

In our research, when Bill and I questioned bulimarexics about their early life, many did report a traumatic loss. However, the descriptions of these losses varied widely. It seems likely that having been asked to search their memories for instances of traumatic loss, these women (or anyone answering this question) might have characterized an event as traumatic that otherwise might not have been viewed as such. For example, one woman mentioned the death of a beloved dog as the trauma that set in motion her binge/purge cycle. Furthermore, these women may have a motivational bias to list instances of traumatic loss as a way of justifying their eating problems. Then there is the problem of studying only individuals who present themselves for treatment, especially chronically ill patients whose starvation may very well skew the results. How do researchers know they are representative? Garfinkle and Garner (1982) concluded it is difficult to make meaningful comments on premorbid personality characteristics as they predispose to anorexia nervosa. In their view, most reports are of limited value since it is very difficult to separate the psychopathological characteristics that are possible precursors of the disorder from those that are by-products of serious illness and are secondary to starvation.

THESE established theories about anorexia die hard and are so entrenched, it is virtually impossible to find any expert in the field who does not adhere to the party line. Socio-cultural rituals and biomedical factors are still viewed as secondary to the severe psychopathology that most researchers associate with the anorexic experience. But as I see it, the cultural mandates of femininity, along with personality traits such as social insecurity, emotional reserve, a deferential, self-denying and self-effacing style, over-compliance, and limited autonomy, are not fixed features of a flawed, anorexic personality but rather a collection of characteristics and compromises all women are socialized to embrace in order to survive and achieve personal and professional success.

In highly significant landmark studies undertaken in the 1970s by Inge Broverman and colleagues, male and female practicing clinicians were given a set of 122 bipolar adjectives, each of which described a behavior trait or characteristic such as very aggressive, not at all aggressive, doesn't hide emotions, always hides emotions, and so on. Their findings suggested that the ideal personality was essentially a masculine model and that women who conformed to the female model were then in the curious position of being normal and deviant at the same time. It was, in fact, impossible to score as both a healthy adult and a healthy woman. The authors observed that so-called feminine traits ran counter to clinical descriptions of maturity and mental health.

When these traits are perceived as pathological, "fixed," and determined, there are serious consequences for treatment. This view reinforces powerlessness and a "therapeutic mystique" that anorexics are biologically and psychologically inferior in significant ways. Think of the implications implicit in diagnosing millions of women as "sick"! This indictment discourages women from participating in social change and encourages them to instead *focus on themselves as the source of their conflicts.*

Susie Orbach (1985) raises an important point about viewing anorexia as "a disorder of puberty." Somehow there is the assumption that there is a world of other teenage girls out there who are all happy, well-adjusted, and dealing quite well with the demands of adolescence. Orbach states: "Behind the notion that this is a disorder of puberty lies another unquestioned assumption. Grown-up femininity is assumed to be unproblematic. The anorexic's refusal to accept her role is, per se, pathological, not an extremely complicated response to a confusing social role" (pg. 129).

Pitfalls Rather than Pathology

Researchers in the field of eating disorders are correct in identifying these traits in anorexics and bulimarexics. Where they err is in viewing them as *pathology* rather than *pitfalls* and studying eating-disordered women in isolation from other women who do not have eating disorders. Psychologist Judith Sills on the *Today Show,* January 1999, has identified several personality pitfalls in her women clients. Women with eating disorders struggle with the same issues:

1. An inability to say "No"
2. Being overly sensitive
3. Being hypercritical (of self and others)
4. Being emotionally dependent (in spite of economic independence)—women need permission to do everything
5. Persistence in clinging to fantasies; i.e., "he'll change."

The danger, of course, is that *pitfalls can become pathology* if the client does not experience an early intervention. Many years of starving and/or bingeing and purging reinforces a "learned helpless" mentality that can mimic immature patterns of behavior and dependency and may cause the client to become more unwilling to give up her symptoms.

The individual pathology model of eating disorders is sexist and destructive and does not answer the questions as to why there are so many women struggling with these problems at this time in history. It does not address the socialization of women for the female role, which Claudia Bebko and Joane Krestan (1990) call the indoctrination into the code of goodness: "Be attractive, be a lady, be unselfish and of service, make relationships work, and be competent without complaint." When millions of women suffer from eating disorders, have low self-esteem, lack self-respect, and do not believe in their capacity to overcome their problems, then we have a global epidemic problem with enormous political implications for treatment. As Naomi Wolf (1985) puts it: "This can no longer be explained as a private issue. If suddenly 60 to 80 percent of college women can't eat, it's hard to believe that suddenly 60 to 80 percent of their families are dysfunctional in this particular way. There is a disease in the air, and its cause was generated with intent and young women are catching it." She challenges us to look at *how society benefits* in much the same way that Betty Friedan (1963) exposed the investment big business had in keeping women at home and consumers in the fifties. Dieting alone constitutes a lucrative $5 to 10 billion industry.

Socio-Cultural Factors that Predispose to Anorexia Nervosa

Let us now move away from the individual/familial pathological model of predisposing factors in eating disorders to one that summarizes social explanations and offers possible social solutions. Researchers Susan Nolen-Hoeksema from University of Michigan and Joan S. Girgus from Princeton University isolated numerous risk factors for depression in adolescence that may also fuel eating disorders. I have borrowed several and added others I feel are relevant. The majority are created by socialization pressures—a process called "gender intensification" that leads girls to adopt some of the following personality characteristics deemed appropriate for their gender: (J. P. Hill and Lynch 1983)

1. Self-esteem becomes based on relationships with others, leading to a conflict of the authentic self with a culturally scripted one that emphasizes "people pleasing"—taking care of everyone else's needs but her own. Taking care of the self is deemed selfish instead of appropriate. In relationships with boys the people pleaser is expected to prevail. Boys are seen as "larger-than-life others" whose needs and feelings take precedence over the girl's needs and feelings. Girls begin to surrender their power, feeling less confident and competent than boys. Typically they come to view a relationship with a boy as critical, often leading to a kind of desperation to have one. Being slim is viewed as absolutely necessary to attract a male. When there is a boyfriend, girls often put aside all of their interests and identities to be available whenever boys expect them to. Rejection is viewed as "catastrophic," and girls blame themselves when things don't work out. These adolescent relationships are rarely equal, so the stage has been set for a "master-slave" mentality that repeats itself

over and over throughout adolescence and often into adulthood as well. Putting too much emphasis on achieving self-worth and self-esteem from relationships puts girls at risk for depression because relationships at this age are not very controllable (Maccoby 1989).

2. Unassertiveness, lack of self-confidence, low expectations for their ability to to control important events. Girls worry about issues of personal worth and being a "good person"; accomplishments and talents are undervalued relative to boys (Coleman 1961; Simmons and Blyth 1987). This leaves them confused about how to achieve self-worth and confidence with a concomitant vulnerability to distress (Nolen-Hoeksema 1995).

3. Negative reinforcement of instrumental skills, talents, intellectual activities, and increased expectation to conform to restrictive social roles deemed appropriate for females. Girls are pressured to pursue feminine gender-typed activities and decrease masculine-typed activities (Gove and Herb 1974).

4. Body-image disparagement and dissatisfaction beginning at a very early age, caused by our fat-phobic cultural values and comparing one's body to the emaciated ideals found everywhere—ideals that are biologically impossible to imitate. Girls worry much more than boys about their appearance.

5. Inadequate coping strategies in the form of a pessimistic attribution style, learned helplessness, a passive ruminative style of coping, and internally focused responses (Nolen-Hoeksema 1995; Nolen-Hoeksema and Girgus, 1994; Sethi and Nolen-Hoeksema 1997).

6. Girls begin to worry much more than boys about personal safety.

All of these same factors and inadequate coping strategies may lead to a desire to lose weight; however, powerful self-perpetuating biological responses of the body to dieting could cause girls *without* these personality risk factors and/or negative life experiences to also develop eating disorders. Since losing weight is now a universal norm and obsession among adolescent girls, we may find—as in breast cancer—that *being female is the major risk factor for developing an eating disorder,* and we may never be able to predict which adolescent girl will convert dieting into the deadly disorder of starvation: anorexia nervosa.

Since there is such an enormous population of women struggling with eating disorders, there is bound to be a cross section of every type of psychiatric illness represented from affective disorders to obsessive-compulsive to borderline personalities—and every type of life experience including sexual abuse and rape. My argument is that the vast majority of eating-disordered women are *brainwashed,* not character disordered and do not evidence serious underlying problems, deficits, or dysfunctional families. Most of the bizarre symptomology goes away with adequate weight restoration.

Each is a unique individual, and their problems and complaints about their families and social life, their fears and fantasies, are no different from other adolescent girls and women I treat for depression and a myriad of other problems. The issues are similar, but the anorexic's method of getting our attention and making a statement—like girls who self-mutilate—is extremely provocative.

In spite of the difficulty in treating anorexics, I have remained incredibly optimistic because the majority of young women I have encountered recover completely without medication or hospitalization, and many respond well to brief (three to six months) episodes of psychotherapy. Therapy can help them achieve a sense of dignity, provide support, help them grow, and handle pain boldly instead of turning it inward against the self. It can help them take risks, assume responsibility, and have equal relationships with others.

These good and deferential females can develop the freedom to identify their true selves, speak their minds and benefit from the realization that we are all in this together. They can learn to express their anger, call themselves women, trust women, redefine what being a woman means, and overcome their eating disorder. I view these girls as having insecurities, anxieties, and self-dissatisfaction—*not* psychosis, *not* personality disorders, *not* developmental deficits that will cripple them forever. I strongly believe that one of the explanations of why men rarely develop eating disorders lies in part in their monopoly in "feeling like a man," which includes being powerful, dignified, and independent: enormous ammunition against feeling worthless, alienated, humiliated, and so on, whereas "feeling like a woman" equals feeling depressed, passive, and all of the characteristics consistently identified in women with eating disorders. As Sanford and Donovan point out in *Women and Self Esteem,* a man who values himself and demonstrates confidence is seen as healthy and normal. But sexual stereotypes are far more restrictive and debilitating for women, so a woman who expresses the same positive self value is condemned as conceited and narcissistic. These catch-22s and double standards define and explain the epidemic of eating disorders. We are socialized to worry excessively and to be humble and self-effacing. Self-denigration and self-hatred are part of the female experience. Until many of the qualities that are synonymous with being a man are also encouraged and embraced by women, an enormous population of young women will continue to become preoccupied with their bodies and attempt to control their appetite whenever personal and social difficulties arise.

Anorexia is another variant of the "feminine mystique"—the potent, hollow promise of the 1950s that trapped women in their homes, relegating them to tasks devalued by society and causing them enormous insecurity, pain, and suffering in the form of fatigue and depression. Betty Friedan called it "the problem that had no name." Anorexia nervosa is a problem that has a name, but it is seen as individually pathological and not collectively political. This has to change. A resurgence of feminist thinking must wrestle the interpretation and treatment of eating disorders from the predominantly medical model.

THREE WOMEN'S STORIES

Listen to these women's stories. Throw away all stereotypical beliefs. Let their true selves shine through, and you will hear women who have enormous strength, phenomenal insights about their episodes of anorexia, and very clear feelings about what helped and did not help in their recovery.

THE following case histories are fairly typical; they are the stories of three current clients who reinforce my argument that prior to dieting, most women who develop eating disorders are *not* biologically nor psychologically inferior in any regard. Michelle, Amy, and Dana were secure, successful, and social, and were more different than they were alike. Two had divorced parents, and for one the breakup was crushing. The third, on the other hand, came from an intact family but disliked her parents and avoided them. In each case, different precipitating factors led to dieting. All became involved in serious episodes of starvation with severe medical implications and while emaciated exhibited classic anorexic thinking and behaviors. Dana recovered on her own, with the help of her family. Michelle stopped starving and purging after a very brief episode of outpatient psychotherapy. But Amy spent an entire summer in a psychiatric hospital and was diagnosed as psychotic and placed on powerful antipsychotic medication because of "one episode." This one episode, according to Amy, was a severe panic attack she experienced after she realized that she was being incarcerated against her will *for the entire summer.* The more agitated she had become after learning the treatment plan, the more severe her restraint and treatment. Amy and her parents, both physicians, had deep misgivings about her diagnosis and medication. So did I after meeting her and hearing her story. In fact, she stopped taking the medication without any consequence. The hospital did succeed in restoring Amy's weight, which in turn facilitated a speedy resolution of her remaining issues. Both Amy and Dana were turned off and resentful of therapists' attempts to force feed them stereotypical explanations of anorexia without letting them have their own voice, their own integrity.

Michelle's Story

Michelle's story underlines the interplay of biological, psychological, and cultural pressures. It illustrates how girls often move from anorexia into bulimarexia and how the two eating disorders can merge and become indistinguishable from each other.

In Michelle's case it was not a negative comment but a positive one that set her eating disorders in motion. She had been swimming a lot at a local health club and had begun to lose weight. Someone commented on it and indicated that she "looked good." She began swimming competitively, practicing four hours a day and cutting out all fat from her diet. Her weight dropped drastically, and more people began commenting about it. She did not see the difference:

I still thought I was fat and continued to exercise and eat very little. My parents made comments on how skinny I was, how I should eat more, and how I was skin and bones, etc. My mom forced me to eat certain foods each morning, and if I didn't she would not allow me to go to swim practice. I ate it reluctantly and felt extremely guilty about the fat I had eaten. After almost two years of doing this, I woke up one morning and blacked out. Doctors told me it was probably because of a lack of body fat, which caused chemical imbalances in my brain and had caused a possible seizure and in turn caused me to black out.

After that incident my mom started buying boxes of Little Debbies, cheesecakes, key lime pies, cookies, and ice cream to make me gain weight. This tactic worked, and I began to gain weight, and by the summer of 1997 at 5'5" I weighed 122 pounds. It may not seem like a lot, but to me I was huge. I hit 122 and freaked. I began taking drastic measures to lose weight. I cut my daily intake of calories to no more than 1,200 calories a day, and I began to exercise constantly. Many days, I ate no more than 800 calories a day and sometimes less than that. I began to take diet pills so I wouldn't feel hungry; I ate just fruit and a sandwich some days. Then after school one day I came home and decided I was hungry. I ate and ate and ate. Leftover pizza, leftovers from dinner, whatever was in the cabinets or refrigerator. After doing this I was overcome with guilt about everything I had eaten, and I tried to make myself throw up. That failed, so I went for the laxatives. I developed a basic pattern. I'd starve myself for a few days, then come home and binge. Then I'd swallow 10–15 laxatives and exercise. I would still feel guilty about doing it, so I'd starve myself again for a few days, and the pattern would start over.

One thing I should mention is the extremely large part my parents played in this. I was extremely unhappy at home (to say the least), and I had never had a good relationship with my family. They were very overprotective, judgmental, and I did not get along with them at all. In a way, by having my eating disorder I was rebelling from them. Problems at home and my eating disorder had been snowballing for almost four years, and one night I simply left my house and didn't go back for weeks. It was obvious that I had a problem and I needed help. I went to my best friend and her mother. When I went to her house that night, it was no intention of mine to tell anyone about my problems, but I ended up talking about it, and now I'm glad I did. My best friend's mother, who I owe so much to, found Dr. White for me, and I am very thankful. I now have new coping skills and better ways to occupy my time. I am doing very well now, and I'm happy to say that I am actually proud of myself. I now have more self-worth, I am taking very good care of myself by eating right and exercising regularly (but not too much). I also think differently now and have a new perspective on things. I have a much happier and positive outlook on everything. I don't hate getting up in the mornings, and I still want to keep living as opposed to many earlier thoughts of suicide. I have rejoined my friends and resumed my social life, which basically came to a complete stop. I will always be extremely cautious about what I eat and taking care of myself, but I am now consciously aware of how to control my eating and how to control other parts of my life in a positive way. I can't say that I will never binge again because I know that it is just setting myself up for failure if I ever do relapse. But hopefully, with the new skills I've learned, and with the help and support of Dr. White, my best friend's mom, and my best friend, I will continue to be strong.

Amy's story is one of unbelievable despair as well as personal triumph. It identifies the classic downward spiral into anorexia and illustrates how anorexia can develop a life of its own, independent from the pressures that gave rise to it.

Amy's Story

I began to lose weight the summer before my junior year of college as part of an effort to become a better cross country runner on my Division III team. I had competed at the national meet the year before, and I was determined to become All-American. I decided the best way to achieve my goal would be to consider myself foremost a runner and to do what the best runners did. This meant no drinking alcohol, running twice a day seven days a week, and never eating junk food. (By junk food I mean the normal definitions: desserts, potato chips, etc.).

I have always had a ravenous appetite, and because I ran in high school, I knew that I could eat as much as I wanted to and remain at 125 pounds (I am 5'6"). So at first I continued to eat a lot, and my running improved. However, as I improved, I lost some weight and began to notice more about the better runners, that they were much smaller and that they were highly disciplined with regard to their running and what they ate. The number-one runner for our team (injured that year because of a pubic bone stress fracture) rarely touched meat, for example, and *never* ate fat. She would eat a big salad (no olives, no dressing) and unbuttered bread, or plain pasta or pasta with marinara sauce, but never anything "sugary" or that contained fat. I also began to be ranked with the Division I girls at the bigger invitational meets, and I was always the biggest girl on the line. I decided to become more stringent, running twice a day seven days a week, doing sit-ups in the mornings and lifting weights in the evenings. I cut out eating meat and fat, and I got positive reinforcement in the form of faster times and positive comments from my coach, who wanted me to convince a few of my teammates to "reform" their eating habits. It is easy not to notice an eating disorder in a sport in which thinness is emphasized. If anyone pointed out that I was getting skinnier, I just pointed out other runners to reassure the person (and myself) that being in training means being lean and cut. I qualified for the national meet again, and I was All-American. The number one girl for our team finished last while wearing a TENS unit for her stress fracture.

It is phenomenal to me now that I didn't realize the vast numbers of runners who are anorexic. My mother was convinced that I was losing too much weight and that the runners to whom I compared myself were "too thin." I dismissed the idea by convincing myself that my mom thought that *everybody* was anorexic and that she just didn't understand that runners have to be skinny. When my high school coach remarked that I was looking "very thin," I thought that my mother had told him that she was afraid I was becoming anorexic. I was surprised to step on the scale and discover that I weighed 111 pounds.

From that point on, I denied that I had a problem. Ironically, the more people mentioned my weight loss, the more defensive I became. I generally was pretty savvy with respect to eating disorders and I knew just how to placate those who pointed out my low weight. I told my high school coach that I loved eating, and I didn't know why I had lost weight—certainly it was not a conscious effort. I told the school doctor that runners have to be thin and compared myself to my other, thinner teammates (yes, there were thinner teammates) who weren't being dragged to the doctor for help with their eating habits. I could generally divert the school counselors attention by talking about the social pressures of being thin (e.g., the evils of *Cosmo* and *Vogue*) and by promising to try to gain weight. I tried to eat conspicuously in front of those of my friends who suspected that I had an eating disorder, and to others who just noticed that I was skinnier, I just said thanks.

Of course, eventually even I couldn't deny "the eating thing," and I was not permitted to run spring track. I was further informed that I would not be permitted to study abroad as I had intended unless I brought my weight up before the spring term. I had to weigh in weekly with the school doctor, and because I had made no progress in gaining weight, she suggested that I not be permitted to go to Germany that spring.

I was appalled that everyone was taking "the eating thing" so seriously, and I convinced my father and the dean of the school to let me go. I told them I was not anorexic, nor afraid to eat or gain weight, and that going to Germany would be the ideal way to appreciate the culture because I could eat whatever I wanted to; I was *supposed* to gain weight.

I had half convinced myself of these things. However, strange things happen to anorexic people. I was afraid to eat certain foods. I didn't realize this until after my recovery. I wouldn't touch peanut butter, for example. To my own mind, I was convinced that I couldn't stand it, although I remembered liking it when I was younger. Chocolate and ice cream? I just didn't see what was special about them. My favorite foods were a nice plain crispy salad, plain popcorn, and a plain baked potato or a baked potato with ketchup. I ate certain soups. I was almost always the last to finish at a restaurant. I wouldn't drink beer because I "didn't want to ruin my training for next season" (four months away). Needless to say, in Germany I didn't exactly put on the weight. I dwindled to 95 pounds, still running daily. On the flight home I tried to order a low-calorie meal.

It seems absurd to me now that I acted this way. I *knew* that I was supposed to gain weight. I was terrified of it, and I didn't know what to do about it. I knew that when the plane touched down, I had to get help. My arrival was disastrous. At the beginning of the trip I had told my father that I was sure I had been gaining weight, so he and my brothers and sister had speculated about what I'd look like arriving at the airport. When I got there they didn't look relieved and happy but afraid. I noticed my sister followed me into the bathroom before we left after exchanging glances with my dad. (They thought I must be bulimic.) I agreed to get help, and after I fainted on the street after a blood test, I spent the week in the heart unit of our local hospital.

My father told me that I could transfer immediately from the hospital to a psychiatric hospital with an eating disorders ward, or I could go home for two weeks first and then go. Of course I didn't want to go, but I knew that I was completely out of control with my eating, and so I agreed to go immediately.

My experience at the eating disorder unit at the psychiatric hospital where I was treated was traumatic. I had spoken to a daughter of one of my friend's fathers who had spent time in two hospitals being treated for her eating disorder. I was aware that the experience had virtually bankrupted her family. My father's friend's daughter spoke very unfavorably of her experience at the hospital into which she was admitted. It did not separate eating disorder patients from other psychiatric patients, had highly restricted visiting, and provided no particular treatment for dealing with problem eating besides consuming the requisite calories. In comparison, the hospital that I was to enter had a relatively small eating-disorders unit. It was reputedly among the top five most successful centers devoted to problem eating in the United States.

Nonetheless, I was completely unprepared for the hospital experience. First, I was convinced that it would take only a few weeks for me to gain back the normal weight outside of the hospital. My illusions were quickly dispelled. Upon entering the hospital, I was astounded to discover that patients had been there for weeks or months and were only too willing to advise me that I would soon get to know the rotations of the menus and become accustomed to the hospital routine. I found the prospect of spending such a long time in the hospital frightening, and I hoped that the length of the other patient's stays were no indication of how long it would take me to gain back the weight.

I remember most of the details of the eating disorders unit itself more vividly than I would prefer to. Foremost, the atmosphere was surreal. The unit itself had about twenty beds, most rooms were doubles, and a large, glass-encased office from which nurses, social workers and psychiatrists could observe the patients. In the center of the common room was a large table were the patients ate and passed the time. There was a television, a washer and dryer, a telephone for ten-minute restricted telephone calls, and a bathroom. Most prominent was the door to the unit, which locked automatically and stood directly underneath a sign warning of the danger to patients trying to flee.

Upon entering the eating disorders unit, my belongings were inspected, and a few items were taken away temporarily and labeled for my use only under supervision: my curling iron, my Walkman, my hair dryer, and any objects that were sharp or had wires. I was told that this was because some patients were at risk for committing suicide, and that I could use my belongings under supervision with my privileges growing as I advanced through certain "stages."

All patients who entered the eating disorders unit were offered a sedative upon entering because the radical change to the hospital environment could be "overwhelming." Everyone that I knew on the unit took the sedatives. Patients were gradually weaned off as the time for discharge approached. Patients were permitted to decline the medication, which I did at first. I took the sedatives later on because I *did* find the atmosphere to be overwhelming.

The new environment was strange and overwhelming for a number of reasons. One thing that anyone entering the unit couldn't help but notice was that one patient, a younger girl in fifth or sixth grade, was never still, but mechanically roamed around the tiny common room, getting up and sitting down several times, energetically pacing the room and repeatedly continuing such behavior. She was chided or gently reprimanded or encouraged not to engage in this behavior by staff and other patients. I was told that calorie-burning activity such as this generally was not to be engaged in except when one advanced to the "stage" in which one could perform supervised aerobics along with a video. The other patients informed me that I would eventually become accustomed to the repetitious activity, and that the girl engaging in it was a special exception to the rule because she had an obsessive-compulsive disorder. One of the older girls told me that this younger girl had accidentally overheard her diagnosis once when the unit's psychiatrist was talking to her parents. According to the older girl, the younger girl had "become" her diagnosis from that time forward and that she engaged in the behavior more when she was particularly distressed.

The first meal at the hospital was unnerving for many. My first experience was not so unnerving, as I did not have to be persuaded to eat. I was informed that patients were allocated one hour during which to complete the meal and that one was not to engage in anorexic behavior, such as abnormal food mixing, cutting one's food into small pieces, or general bad manners, if one could help it. There were nurses who observed all of the patients by sitting at the head of the table and watching the patients eat so that no patient attempted to hide food. There was also a rule that new patients had to remain in the common room to be observed for one hour following meals so that there would be no chance of purging after meals. Bathroom excursions were also supervised (door open, no stall), until one had passed through the requisite "stages." Furthermore, patients' hands had to remain on the table at all times. We listened to music when we ate: Pachalbel's Canon in D for the first several weeks that I was a patient. The song still reminds me of the hospital.

I was congratulated on my good behavior during my first meal and told that if one didn't complete a meal within the requisite time, she got three "warnings" and then would be intubated and force-fed. Naturally, we were all terrified of this. I did notice that patients occasionally exhibited compassion toward one another as if there were solidarity against the oppressive eating disorders unit policies. I particularly remember a new patient who could not face eating her first meal. She was very young and burst into tears upon both her first and second meals and could not finish. At the third meal, when she looked exasperatedly at the tray of food, another patient, who was my age, finally spoke to her. She told the girl it wasn't her fault, "they" [the hospital] were making all of us eat, patients had no say in the matter, they were being forced against their wills, etc. I was astounded that not a single nurse or social worker spoke up. I was terrified of engaging in any behavior that might be construed as noncompliant, and to me this speech seemed insurrectionist and indicated that the staff was unfeeling. However, the speech was effective, the patient finished eating, and the nurses said nothing.

Sometimes I think that the hospital experience would not have been so bad if it weren't for the lack of explanation for the stringent rules to which we had to adhere. Some patients had many more privileges than others. Some patients could spend time outside, go on small excursions— such as group trips to the zoo or the park—and got to eat at the cafeteria, selecting their food through the regular cafeteria line rather than a week in advance from a menu, as the rest of us did. I was completely frustrated throughout my stay because it seemed to me that my advancement through the "stages" moved at a glacial pace. I will always relish sunshine a little more than the general population, I think, because that is what I craved the most during the first four or five weeks at the hospital. When I was finally permitted to go outside, supervised with a social worker for a ten-minute excursion to sit on the lawn outside the hospital, I was so happy that I cried. One overlooks pleasures like feeling the natural heat of sun or experiencing brightness of light until the time when one is deprived of such experiences. Anyway, now I make sure to get outside for a little sunshine and some exercise every day, regardless of the weather.

Only later did I learn that the reason that patients were confined without "privileges" for so long was that there was a real risk of recalcitrant patients running away, the staff were not enough in number to supervise excursions, and hypermetabolism put new patients at a significant risk of significant weight loss if they walked or moved around too much. However, the hospital staff did not apprise patients of these reasons. Furthermore, some obviously skinnier patients moved through the stages more rapidly than others. It seemed so oppressive and arbitrary to me that I had been in the hospital for such an unbearably long time "making no progress," while others quickly advanced through the stages and were even discharged when they obviously were skinnier and in some cases not committed to recovery. In the meantime, I ate meals of Herculean portions and was powerless to advance. (At one time, I was eating three regular meals and two "snacks" per day, in addition to four Hershey bars to supplement and two half-cup "power shakes," designed to pack in extra calories.) I eventually learned that there were two ways to advance through the stages: (1) gain the weight, (2) exhaust your insurance policy. Because of the rules regarding confidentiality of insurance coverage, health care workers, in fairness, *could not* explain why some patients advanced more quickly than others. However, to a group of patients who tensely awaited the periodic review board meetings, and whose progress was not expedited by the emergency conditions of being discharged with no coping skills whatsoever due to lapsed insurance, the reports of the meetings were an occasion to be dreaded.

Additionally, one had to undergo the harrowing experiences of edema associated with weight gain (special socks were issued), the taking of a suppository common during the initial refeeding period, the Metamucil "cocktail" that accompanied our garantuan meals, and weight stagnancy, about which we could do nothing. Together, these experiences coupled with the strict rules of conduct and lack of explanation when patients felt desperate and hopeless. The times that I most relished were when I could talk on the telephone to the real world, visits from my family, and playing cards with the young social workers, who treated patients like people. Anyone entering the hospital should do all they can to gather such outside support before entering because such contact is unbelievably helpful for one's morale.

Furthermore, there is a happy ending to most patients' stays in the hospital. The obsessive-compulsive patient grew out of her obsessiveness when her family or friends visited, and some of the patients keep in touch after their release. I still exchange yearly Christmas cards with my best friend from the hospital.

The ten weeks I spent at the hospital were very unpleasant, and I still don't like to dwell on the wasted summer that I spent there. Many times people said, "But it's not wasted time; getting over anorexia will make you stronger." This still seems silly to me. However, the hospital did for me what no one else could: It helped me to gain the weight back.

I consider my real recovery to have occurred in my senior year of college, when I returned to school at my normal weight. I still thought of some things the way an anorexic person would. I occasionally hated weighing what I did, I thought I looked fat in some of my clothes, I preferred not to eat out, I was really afraid of *wanting* to eat. However, having been in the hospital for approximately ten weeks, I emerged able to estimate the precise calorie content of any portion of a variety of foods. I also knew the precise number of calories that would keep me at my target weight, provided I didn't run. (I was advised to add about 200 calories per mile of running.) Knowing this information, I could maintain my weight. I gave myself no choice but to obey the hospital's recommendations. I had to attend therapy once a week with Dr. White, I had to eat the requisite calories, I could not compete on the cross country or track teams, I had to remain in my target weight range: 123–127 pounds.

I have never really been a big fan of therapy, which is probably why I get along well with Dr. White. This is not to say that Dr. White does not engage in very effective therapy. Dr. White concentrates on solving problems. She understands the anorexic mindset, which is (as I experienced it): "I'll be happy to do anything, so long as it doesn't involve gaining weight or eating." My goal was to maintain my weight that year. I ended up overcoming anorexia.

Prior to my hospitalization, I had talked to several counselors. They said things like, "You're perfectionistic; try not to be hard on yourself; you have low self-esteem; you overemphasize the importance of appearance," etc. They said that anorexics are never *cured,* they are always *recovering* from a food-restricting addiction. They said that in all likelihood, I would always be worried about my weight but that the good news was that I probably would never become overweight. Some of them took a "Mr. Rogers" approach, talking about feelings, pressures, etc. At the hospital, I was given various tests with questions that were characteristic of anorexics. Some were predictable ("Are you involved in cheerleading, running, gymnastics?"); some were surprising ("Do you play golf?"). I also read about anorexia, trying to learn why I became anorexic. I fit some of the stereotypes: involved in a sport emphasizing thinness, alcoholism in my family, upper-income family. Other stereotypes really baffled me: My parents are not authoritative—on the contrary, they are notably permissive; I was never pressured to compete in sports or to work on my appearance. I was completely frustrated at the idea that I didn't know what made me the way I was and that even if I ever found out, the best I could hope for would be recognition of the triggering factors; I could never overcome the anorexia.

Dr. White does not believe in self-victimization. She takes an objective look at what is causing the immediate problem. She then tells her patients to implement the changes and report back. It absolutely works. I have worked on several problems with Dr. White. For example, shortly after returning to school, I was fearful of exceeding my daily calorie allowance because I was hungry. Unlike most other anorexics, I *knew* that I would be eating extra calories and that extra qualities caused extra weight. I was spartan about sticking to my eating schedule until I decided to confess my fear at therapy. Dr. White was entirely reasonable. I began to see that eating an extra apple (or, as Dr. White suggested, an extra piece of cake) would not make me fat, it would not make me gain a pound (unless done habitually). Even if I gained a pound (or, as Dr. White suggested, five pounds), people probably wouldn't notice. Even if I gained ten or twenty pounds, I could take the weight off. No one would force me to be overweight! After I listened to Dr. White's reasoning, I began to understand that eating an extra apple was really not such a big deal. There was a hitch: After concurring in the logic that eating an extra apple is "not catastrophic" (Dr. White's favorite words), I had to agree that if I was hungry and wanted an extra apple, I'd eat it, see what happened, and report back.

I'd like to be able to say that there was an apocalyptic moment when I bit into an apple and realized that I didn't have to answer to anyone (even my anorexic conscience) about what I ate or how I looked, but that's not how it happened. I got hungry and I ate an apple. We never had another therapy session about eating extra food. (I'm smiling as I write this, having just eaten an extra bowl of oatmeal, despite having skipped running today because of inclement weather. I think I'll survive.)

All of this is to say: Don't despair; you can overcome an eating disorder. I'll freely admit that I don't always drink real Coke; in fact, I usually order diet. I also still take things a little more seriously than I probably should. But I am not afraid to ask for help, I don't cringe when I go out to eat anymore, and I will never worry about an extra apple (or an extra piece of cake!). After being two years out of therapy, I am seeing Dr. White again to help me learn how to handle stress now that I'm a second-year law student. I don't worry about becoming addicted to therapy any more. Dr. White helps people to solve their own problems: Her goal is to get you over the problem and get you out of therapy. People can change the way they react, behave, and think about things. Anorexics don't have to live according to their diagnosis.

Finally, when I was anorexic, I used to think to myself, What a thankless job to deal with anorexics who are trying to recover. They are irritable and push away people who try to help them. If I had an anorexic audience at arm's length, this is what I would say:

You have to gain the weight. All the weight. I promise that you will feel better, but you have to gain the weight—you won't cheat anyone but yourself if you don't. And you have to do it first. Talking won't help until you gain the weight.

People die from anorexia. Anorexia causes bone loss, hair loss; it makes your hands cold. Your organs, especially your heart, can be irreparably damaged. Anorexia harms your metabolism. Anorexia is dangerous; people are right to be worried about it.

You can overcome anorexia. Get help. Your parents and friends are not enough. (It's too easy to dismiss their advice because they are who they are.) You need someone to be a parole officer and a cheerleader. There are people who aren't fascinated by anorexia and who understand it and who can help you. Life is too short to worry about the extra apple.

Dana's story does seem to reinforce the traumatic-loss theory. She had several psychosocial stressors that were devastating, including the divorce of her parents and a move to a new environment. However, dieting occurred after a long period of torment in which she was teased unmercifully about being "chubby." Like the others, dieting turned into full-blown anorexic symptoms and behaviors. These symptoms began to disappear as she gained weight, and her body-image disparagement ceased after a short period of nutritional rehabilitation. Both Dana and Amy are currently in therapy with me. As Amy related, she has completely overcome anorexia, is now a second-year law student, and recently returned to therapy to work on stress-reduction strategies—our conversations have nothing to do with eating or food. Dana is also presently in therapy for help with some of her oppositional/defiant self-defeating behaviors. She is decidedly not the proverbial "good girl." She too has completely overcome her bout with anorexia, has no desire to diet, and we have never had to deal with this issue in therapy.

Dana's Story

I grew up in a very stable household, with a mother, father, and an older brother. My parents were both very devoted to my brother and I and always spent plenty of time with us. We grew up in a safe neighborhood and went to a small local public school. I had several hobbies such as animals, and I loved to write. My grades were mostly A's, and occasionally I would get a few B's. I had a couple of very close friends and many friendly acquaintances. My future was stable, in my mind, and I had a few very strong goals I wanted to achieve. Life was good.

During my 6th grade year in middle school, my parents separated. I was completely devastated. I remember knowing instinctively that my life was going to be changed forever by this, yet I had resolved to take things in stride. I would continue doing well in school, go on to high school, and visit my father on the weekends whenever I could. I somehow made it seem tolerable for a while . . . then I received another shock: My mother met another man, and he lived all the way in Virginia. She eventually decided to move down there to be with him, and I was very unhappily taken along. My mother thought it make sense for me to be with her and for my brother to stay with my father; to her it seemed to be the most reasonable and fair thing to do. To me it was the worst thing anyone could ever do to me, and I spent many weeks begging and pleading for her to let me stay where I was. Ultimately, though, she had the upper hand in the decision. We packed up our things and loaded up the green Taurus with our necessities, and I reluctantly watched my brother and father grow farther and farther away until I couldn't see them any longer.

All of a sudden I was petrified. My entire life had been uprooted and was about to be replanted in, what was my opinion, poisonous soil. I thought we might move in to some trashy, two-room apartment on West 31st Street or something. Everyone at my new school, I thought, was going to be a bunch of gangsters. My stepsisters were going to be evil, like in the movie *Cinderella*. I no longer had the protection of my older brother. I felt exposed, vulnerable, and scared for the first time in my life. The worst part was that I knew my mother was just as scared as I was. When my mother and her boyfriend, Gary, were first together, he lived across town in a two-family apartment, and she and I lived in a small brick ranch near a "good school." They spent a lot of time together in the afternoons and on weekends, and then I met his children. He had a 12-year old, Dawn, and an 8-year old, Ashley, at the time; I was also 12. On the weekends we would all go hiking or swimming or to an amusement park. They had us do a lot of fun things, and tried their best to make us happy about the whole situation. Dawn and I became very close since we were the same age and we were both going through the same thing. We soon became inseparable and wanted to do everything together all the time. I would beg my mom to let her come over, which she didn't mind because then she could spent time with her boyfriend. Dawn was a lot skinnier than I was. I had always been on the chubbier side but never stressed about it too much. I had also never had a "real" boyfriend before, but Dawn talked about guys a whole lot, and my attention went from animals and writing stories to the hot guys in the red jeep. A lot of times we would go swimming at the beach or a public pool, and I would feel self-conscious next to her because she was a lot thinner, and guys would always look at her. She was also very pretty. I thought I was pretty, too, but ugly in comparison to her. I began to obsess about my weight. At my new school, I got teased about being chubby a lot more than I ever had before. I remember one boy said "Hey, try Weight Watchers!" when I walked onto the school bus. I was mortified. During the school day I was always self-conscious in class, and I didn't have any friends. All my friends were back at home. I would either sit alone at lunch or with the weird group of kids, the outcasts. When I wasn't feeling low in school, I was at home feeling low. I would go home after school, before my mom got home from work, and eat almost a whole bag of tortilla chips—I wasn't even hungry, and I didn't really like chips, I just zoned out and ate them. Every weekend that Dawn and Ashley came to our house to visit, Dawn would tease me about being chubby. She wasn't intentionally trying to hurt me, but it stung every time she said something about my weight. I kept telling myself for months that I would go on a diet, but it wasn't until the summer that I had finally had enough.

A lot of the time during the summer me, my mom, Gary, Dawn, and Ashley were doing something new and exciting. We went to water parks, hikes, beaches, picnics, etc. My brother also came down to visit for a few weeks, and it would be Dawn and I in the way-back seat of the Taurus, my brother and Ashley in the middle seats, and mom and Gary in the front. At first, I didn't give too much thought to dieting; it was just that my mind was preoccupied with other things: guys, being popular, and my new best friend. A lot of times Dawn and I would walk off from the rest of the family because we were "too cool" for them. Ashley would try and tag along a lot, but we left her out more than we let her come along. Soon, however, I found myself wanting to eat less and less. During an entire day at the water park, for instance, all I would eat would be maybe an orange and a lot of soda to keep me full. If my mother packed sandwiches for everyone, I would ask her to make me a cucumber sandwich. I would eat the cucumbers and throw away the bread when no one was looking. At night, I would skip dinner as much as I could get away with it. It wasn't long before I noticed a change in my body. My stomach was flatter, and my thighs were slimmer. Plus I had a nice summer tan to go along with it. It soon became addictive, it was almost a high. I felt lightheaded and hungry a lot, but I became used to the feeling and almost enjoyed it. Once I went the entire day eating only an apple, and another time I only drank juice all day. I did make a friend up the street from me, and one day she and I went bike riding. I became so lightheaded and cranky that I slammed my bike down in frustration. She kept asking me what was wrong, and I just said I needed to lie down and told her to go home. It took all my energy to go back inside the house and lie down on my bed. I wouldn't ever let anyone else make my food for me because I was paranoid that they might try to pour butter on it when I wasn't looking. My mom tried to cook me healthy, low-fat dinners, but I would look at them and "see" butter in them when they were really just water droplets. Of course, I got feedback from other people around me. One day while I was walking my dog, my next-door neighbor said, "Wow, what did you do? You look like you've lost so much weight!" To me that translated to, "You still need to lose a few more pounds, and then you'd look perfect." In reality, I realize now that it probably meant, "Wow you lost a lot of weight really fast, are you sick? You look too skinny." At that time, I probably weighed about 120 pounds, which is a good weight for my height, 5′3″. But my fear of gaining it back is what kept me from eating normally. One morning Dawn and I were getting dressed and she turned around and looked at me and said, "Oh, my gosh, look at you, you've got curves! You don't need to lose any more weight, please don't. I'm worried about you." Her concern only added fuel to the fire. Hearing that from the one person who teased me so much enraged me, but I kept it all inside, and resolved never to eat again.

Near the end of the summer, my mom was so concerned about me that she decided to send me to a therapist. I was open-minded about it; I knew I had some sort of problem, but I didn't think anyone was going to help me. During the first session the lady asked me why I decided to go on a diet, and I told her simply because I was chubby and wanted to lose weight. She basically contradicted what my reasons were, and told me no, there was some other "underlying" reason for my anorexia. She suggested that maybe since my parents were divorced, I felt out of control, and so I started trying to control myself instead. I was asked if I had been sexually abused. Then the lady told me I was never really fat, I was just a normal-sized teenager for my age but I *thought* I was fat. I didn't like how she stereotyped me from the moment I walked in there. It was almost like she had some hidden list somewhere that she studied called "Theories for Anorexia." In a way she was right. The reason was because my life had been changed so drastically, and suddenly I was in a world where the pressures to be thin outweighed most everything else. That world is called society.

Most of the time that I went to see a specialist or a therapist, I felt like they were regarding me as a sick person, someone they had to tiptoe around and touch lightly in case I might break. Even my mother didn't know what to do with me, and she tried everything. At that time I was frustrated with everyone. I was tired of being labeled and put into a category. The first time someone called me "anorexic" I was shocked. That name did not belong to me. The more people tried to help, the more it agitated me because in a way, they were the ones who caused it in the first place. Most likely they did it unintentionally, but I felt like I couldn't trust anyone. That is when I started showing signs of obsessive-compulsive behavior. My grades in school the following year were straight A's. My handwriting was absolutely perfect. I kept my room completely spotless and organized. I was conscious of what I was doing the entire time, but I didn't know why I did it. It would amuse me when people tried to diagnose, explain, or treat my behavior. If *I* didn't know exactly why I was doing it, how would *they* know?

I did know for sure that I was homesick beyond belief. I just wanted to go back and live with my dad and brother and see my old friends again. I knew deep down inside that things would somehow be better if I moved back there. At first, my mother resisted, but eventually she gave in because it was the last thing she could try to help me get better. During January of my 7th grade year, my father drove down to Virginia in a moving van to come and get me. Not much was said as we packed up the van with my things, and Gary held on to my mom as I waved good-bye with hardly a smile. The whole drive back up to Massachusetts was a quiet one; I didn't say too much to my dad, and he didn't push me to say anything either. I knew he was overjoyed to have me home, and he knew that I was relieved and content again. Waves of relief washed over me when I saw the familiar northern pine trees and felt the cold sting of Massachusetts weather. When we pulled into our driveway, I was greeted by my brother and his new girlfriend, and they helped me and Dad unload the van. My brother didn't say much to me, either; he just gave me a big long hug and smiled at me.

At first my dad was scared because I wasn't showing any improvement. My weight at that time was 102 pounds, dangerously low. I knew, though, that I was going to be OK. He threatened to send me to the hospital if I didn't start to eat soon. Yet at the same time he was very patient with me and gave me space and time to recuperate. One day I ate a bowl of cereal in front of him. I acted real nonchalant, like I had been doing it all along, but I think his eyes popped out of his head. It took me a long time, and at first I really didn't eat, I only drank soda. I pretty much reversed the process. Then I went through a phase where I would only eat one meal a day, and it would always be rice and beans. I even let my dad put the amount of food he thought I should eat on my plate as long as I got to supervise the cooking of the food. No butter or oil was ever allowed. As my appetite started coming back, I was constantly ravenous. I was worried that I would gain too much weight, but I forced myself to look at myself realistically, and no matter how much I ate, I only gained a little back. Finally my perception came back to normal. One day I remember looking in the mirror and thinking that my arms looked like one of those starving Somalians. I was disgusted that I actually treated my body like that, and for what? The only boyfriend I had was in early 7th grade, and he dumped me because he said I never talked or did anything. Hello?! I was starving to death; I couldn't see straight; how could that be attractive to a guy?

I think a lot of young girls are given the wrong messages. When they are twelve and thirteen, they're not grown yet, but they're not kids anymore, either. At that age they distance themselves from their parents, and they are not old enough to be on their own and handle everything well, but yet they are too old to be under the protection of their parents all the time. That's the situation I was in, along with the pressures of adjusting to a new school, new family, and new friends. At that age girls no longer see things from their parents' modified point of view but from their own. The importance to be socially accepted is magnified one thousand times while at the same time the importance to be accepted by family decreases. Instead of being around people who love and appreciate them for who they are, they suddenly find themselves around people who are there for reasons other than love. I thought I would be alone for the rest of my life if I didn't lose weight. The only thing I really needed to do was to gain confidence.

10.

Intensive Psychotherapy with Anorexics

BEGINNING THERAPY

In the 1980s treating anorexics on an outpatient basis was less demanding because most were first referred to inpatient eating-disorder programs for weight restoration. This was my standard procedure, in spite of deep misgivings over the authoritarian and often coercive behavior-modification treatment they received, forced to eat and gain weight in intense power struggles with their doctors. A prominent English psychiatrist, Dr. P. J. Dally, expressed this view: "When encountered in its extreme form, these patients are formidable adversaries, giving and expecting no mercy. The doctor may falter and quail, compromising with them, and in effect allowing them to dominate their treatment and continue their downward path unchecked. To succeed with these clients a doctor must be as ruthless as they are, confine them to bed and force them to obey" (1979).

Yet however miserable and contentious the hospital stay, it was easier to begin outpatient treatment with a client like Amy who had gained ten or fifteen pounds, was no longer in medical danger, and was feeling more alert and energetic after nutritional rehabilitation. Today, unless the client is close to death and/or in need of drastic medical intervention, her HMO will typically refuse to certify her for inpatient care. It is a worrying picture. Where are all of these starving girls receiving treatment? Only a handful of eating-disorder programs are still surviving. Managed-care companies are invested in cutting costs, substituting drug therapy for psychotherapy, and developing contracts with less credentialed providers who will accept lower fees. Since both inpatient and outpatient resources are now so meager, I shudder to think of the enormous human and economic toll as this deadly epidemic continues to expand.

Before a client's first session, I require an initial medical evaluation to make sure she can safely be seen on an outpatient basis. There is not much sense initiating therapy with a client who is in need of immediate hospitalization. This evaluation will diagnose coexisting medical problems as well as establish the severity of malnutrition. Hopefully the physicians will also discuss with the client the physical dangers of her behaviors. Each client may have a different primary care physician (PCP), so it is important to build bridges and dialogue with a number of local physicians.

Once the PCP gives the go-ahead to treat the client, we then discuss follow-up medical management as well as nutritional rehabilitation. Each doctor has a preferred format. If the client is emaciated, she might need to be seen weekly. Other clients return to their PCPs monthly. Unless one works in a hospital setting or large clinic, it is no longer possible in private practice to separate weight restoration from psychotherapy. Prior to managed care, my physician consultant handled weighing clients and monitoring their weight gain. This freed me to participate in a more nurturing/trusting empathetic role. This too is no longer possible, so our initial consultation must determine whether or not the client can and will meet the expected goal of weekly weigh-ins and restoration of normal weight at a minimal rate of one-half to one pound per week. Psychotherapy without weight restoration and nutritional rehabilitation is simply not effective. It must go hand in hand with them, which places new demands on the therapist. I had to become extremely well educated about nutrition, the side effects of starvation, exercise physiology, how much to eat—the hows, whats, wheres, and whens—set point, resting metabolism, triggers of disinhibited eating, and so on.

The therapist must talk about food and process the client's fears of eating, gaining weight, feeling full, and becoming fat as well as confidently deflect irrational phobic beliefs about these issues in a soothing, reassuring manner, emphasizing facts about nutrition. The client must feel she is with a wiser, smarter person than herself and come to trust and ultimately believe the evidence the therapist presents to counter her own uneducated conclusions. Later, the nutritional consultant will provide expert backup and assume some of the burden of nutritional counseling. However, typically at this early stage the client will not benefit from a nutritional consultation.

The first few sessions with an anorexic are a much different experience from those with bulimics. The latter wants help, hates what she is doing, and is deeply ashamed of her lack of control. The anorexic is under the influence of starvation and is often depressed, irritable, apathetic, and in major denial about the seriousness of her condition. Usually she is pressured to come to therapy against her will. She is not happy to be there and just wants everyone to leave her alone. Anorexic clients best suited for outpatient treatment are those who are not severely emaciated but in the beginning stages and do not require inpatient hospitalization. Anorexic clients who are leaving inpatient programs and need intensive follow-up are also good candidates.

The first sessions are designed to: learn about the client's history and family, her wishes, and her dreams; establish rapport and begin a therapeutic alliance; clearly delineate the rules and goals of therapy; and begin to educate the client about the impact of starvation on her body. I do not entertain any preconceived notions, embrace any theories, any expectations. I want to know who this unique person is—what she is like under the starving body and baggy clothes. I like to spend time alone with both the family and the client during the first sessions. (Subsequent sessions are also solo or family sessions, depending on each client's particular situation.) They know her better than anyone else and are desperate to help and get help for themselves. I want them to know how I work, what my values and expectations are, and the rules and goals of therapy. I want them to feel comfortable, and I encourage questions. I need them on my side, and I also need to know about their prior therapy experiences, their values, what interventions they have tried. What has worked and what has not worked? I want them to express their feelings, as I want to support their efforts and understand their pain.

Most parents I encounter are completely devastated and demoralized by what they have read in the literature, which often paints them as interfering with their daughter's autonomy—weakening her reliance on her own thoughts, emotions, perceptions, and behaviors—and reinforces the belief that her functioning is inherently deficient. Parents are said to be "clinically ill" in their discouragement of their child's self-reliance while rewarding compliance (Masterson 1977).

Although troubled families of course exist, I have rarely encountered parents like the ones described. More often I see people who need help and guidance and do not know what to do. Typically they are good, caring people who have tried heroically on their own to love their child out of her problem. They are very afraid, with good reason, that their daughter might die. Eventually everything they do seems wrong. Rather than indict them, *therapy must provide a problem-solving, solution-based collaborative atmosphere of mutual respect.* Every session should be an opportunity to look at what happened the previous week and what problems have been encountered. The parents need to participate fully and feel they are part of the healing, not the cause of the problem.

During the initial intake session, the client is asked to fill out two inventories. One is a standard psycho-social assessment, and the other is an eating-disorder evaluation of my own construction. Written responses are encouraged via questions that elicit more than yes and no answers, questions that may lead to other insights about the client such as: "If a movie were made about your life, what would the title be?"

In my inventory I want to find out how the client viewed her life prior to her decision to diet. What is she satisfied and dissatisfied with, and what would she like to change? Have there been any traumas, conflicts, major problems? What does she see as her strengths and weaknesses? What is her attitude/motivation to gain weight, make changes, and be in therapy? How does she view her social life, friends, family? Does she feel she has any support? What does she do for fun? Whom does she respect? I read these evaluations carefully in order to create an individualized treatment plan. This is an important point because it is critical that each client be evaluated for her own issues, *not for anorexia.* As we have seen, many clients have expressed their anger, resentment, and frustration at being categorized, labeled, and interpreted via "the theory." Many times the therapist *told* them what their problems were and threw some of the typical explanations for the disorder at them such as, "You feel like a failure and that you have no control in your life and this is your way of gaining some feelings of accomplishment." While there may be some truth to this, each client needs to be allowed to *tell her own story,* expressing her own individuality and understanding of how she got into such a fix. If the reason is serendipity—for example, a diet gone crazy—it is not useful for the therapist to keep fishing for deeper underlying issues.

Since a great deal of relevant information is compiled during the initial sessions, developing rapport, trust, and respect then becomes the immediate focus. A basic step is to assess whether or not a collaborative working relationship is possible. The first few sessions are a process of mutual discovery and evaluation. I will do almost anything to get anorexics to talk to me. (My first job after graduate school was spent at a residential treatment facility for troubled adolescents in upstate New York. For five years I struggled with learning how to talk to hostile and/or nonverbal adolescents. It was good experience for my later work with anorexics. I will often share personal experiences and discuss my values and avocational interests. I encourage the girls to ask questions, and I answer them as honestly as possible even if I know the client will not like the answer. It is not my style to be superaffectionate like Peggy Claude-Pierre or to have a nurturant-authoritative approach like Stephen Levenkron, the author of *The Best Little Girl in the World.* My work differs from client to client and session to session, depending on the needs, attitudes, and experiences of the client. If a client has worked hard that week and gained weight, I want to be very reinforcing and positive. If she is exhibiting resistance, I may employ "tough-love" strategies or gentle encouragement.

Establishing Rapport

My approach in the first session alone with the client might go something like this:

I know it is difficult for you to be here, and you probably would rather be elsewhere, but today we have the very important job of determining if you can safely be treated on an outpatient basis without disrupting your life or if you will need to be hospitalized and receive treatment there. *You have everything to say about which option you choose.* I would really prefer the first—that we work hard together to help you overcome this problem without taking you away from school, home, and friends. This certainly will be one of the hardest jobs you have ever undertaken, but I hope it will become one of the things you will be the most proud of as well! In your life, you will look back and value things that have been the most difficult. You don't need help when things are easy, right? Overcoming anorexia demands a lot of character, honesty—with yourself and others—and a real fighting spirit. I would not do this work if people did not recover. I would not spend my time watching people deteriorate.

You have probably read a lot about anorexia and may or may not agree with the way this problem is interpreted and how anorexics are characterized. I would like to throw all of this away and not generalize anything about you. I want to get to know you as an individual with your own unique issues and not put you into a neat little anorexic box. The majority of the many girls and women that I have treated are more different than they are alike. *I view starvation as the problem.* That is the most important thing we have to tackle. You are going to have to gain weight—this is inevitable, and it will be a very hard road. It is my job to help you deal with all of your "dragons"—your fears and fantasies about weight gain, your worrying about gaining too much weight, your feelings of fullness, and so on. I know a lot about this problem. I promise you that you will be able to handle what is expected, and I hope you will learn to trust me. *I promise you will not gain too much weight.* I will help you with this. It is going to be a lot more difficult to gain weight than you believe.

Your thinking has become screwy, and a lot of this is *not your fault.* You are under the influence of starvation and *you will feel better, not worse, as you begin to gain weight.*

Rules, Goals, and Education

At this point, psychoeducational material related to the effects of starvation is introduced. The PCP's medical findings are discussed as well as information from Professor Ancel Key's studies on starvation (mentioned in Chapter 6) as they relate to the clients medical symptoms. The client is shown how her symptoms of fatigue, irritability, apathy, depression, poor concentration, and social isolation are connected to her malnourishment. The rules and goals of therapy are reiterated, with honesty a number-one requirement! Some therapists weigh their clients backward and do not specify a target weight goal—on the assumption that the client will not be able to handle it or will become overly obsessed with the results. My preference is to show the client her progress and deal with her anxiety about it during the therapy session. There is some evidence that exposure to weight gain is actually associated with the reduction in the fear of gaining weight (Morgan and Russell 1975).

Dos and don'ts for parents are negotiated in these initial sessions with inappropriate expectations identified. For example, pushing the anorexic to eat ice cream or hamburgers is not helpful in the beginning stages of therapy. We work on a food plan, and I often recommend supplements such as Slim Fast as a way of obtaining additional calories. Slim Fast is more appealing to clients (for obvious reasons) than nondiet supplements such as Ensure. Supplements are useful because the amount of food the anorexic must eat in order to gain the appropriate weight is substantial, usually a minimum of 3,000 calories a day, which makes an already difficult process even more traumatic. Clients are reassured that they can discontinue the supplements when they achieve a healthy weight.

The target weight goal needs to be agreed upon as soon as possible. A goal weight range of three to five pounds above the client's weight threshold to maintain menstruation, and approximately 10 percent below her highest weight prior to the onset of the disorder, is a good yardstick to start with. A recent study of one hundred anorexics in the *Archives of Pediatrics and Adolescent Medicine* (January 1997) concluded that a return of menses occurred after achieving a weight approximately 90 percent of the previous standard body weight prior to starvation. Another study by researchers at Massachusetts General Hospital found weight gain, not estrogen replacement, improved bone density.

Other factors also play a part in determining a target weight range. With a client who had inappropriate eating habits and/or did not exercise prior to the dieting attempt, it may be possible for her to be thinner than 10 percent of her highest weight if she will commit to a conscientious food plan and a moderate, nonobsessive exercise program. For example, if Sara's highest weight was 135 pounds at 5′4″ tall, and she ate a lot of junk food and never exercised, it might be possible for her to achieve a weight of 125 pounds instead of 135 pounds. However, caution is in order, for in my experience many of the clients who relapse are those who have overcome starvation but who continue trying to maintain a suboptional weight that is biologically impossible. Flexibility on the part of the therapist and experimentation on the part of the client are often necessary. I also ask parents to bring in pictures of their daughter prior to her recent weight loss to evaluate how she looked at her highest weight. The therapist must explain why it is impossible for the client to weigh whatever "ideal" weight she has chosen and why one cannot just pick out a particular celebrity such as Calista Flockhart and decide to weigh what she does. The genetics of metabolism, body composition, and set point are all explained, and special attention is given to a discussion of critical weight: the level of body fat necessary for the resumption of menses. When anorexics envision "fat," they imagine it as grease dripping and/or as globs attached to their hips or stomach, not as a protective internal layer. We talk how their body has been dangerously cannibalizing itself—using up protein muscle to maintain fuel for their energy needs—and how this process could lead to irreversible long-term consequences such as osteoporosis and infertility.

They are reassured that their body "knows" where the weight they gain needs to go to. It knows where muscle is needed, when the kidneys need a thicker layer of fat for protection, and so on. Food is reinforced as *fuel and medicine,* not as the enemy to be feared. We discuss how they looked and how they ate prior to their starvation episode. We examine the pictures their parents brought in. They are given honest feedback with an emphasis on remembering how normal, satisfied, and unafraid they were about eating and their bodies before they began dieting. If they looked slightly chubby, we discuss how they could have handled it in a healthy, nutritionally sound manner.

Strategies for consuming the necessary calories for weight gain are processed with the client having the final word about how and in what form (supplements, snacks, larger meals) she is willing to commit to. The clients are weighed once a week on the clinic scale and are instructed not to weigh themselves on any other scales at any other time. Plateaus and occasional glitches are tolerated, but major weight loss of any type is presented as *totally unacceptable.*

When requested, I will hand out a food plan with many choices from a famous health spa—where the "stars" go to lose weight. Although the food plan is only 1,200 calories, it serves to reinforce the fact that these clients are consuming far fewer calories than the spa diet allows. It is a reassuring place to start, though I always have to carefully explain to parents why I am giving their daughter a "diet." Starting with the 1,200 calories, gradual weekly increases lead up to the 3,000 calories a day that is needed for weight gain.

Anorexic rituals and games such as cooking for everyone else, eating separate meals, and not eating with the family are immediately eliminated. Clients are expected to keep a daily food diary, which they bring to each session for discussion. The family often participates as observers. Individual work with the client occurs as the parents look on, and we also engage in family therapy where questions are raised and problems addressed. Individual sessions are also conducted as needed. Exercise is usually initially disallowed. As the client begins to gain weight, with the physician's approval, minimal supervised muscle-bearing exercise may be approved. Allowing anorexics to engage in muscle-bearing activity once they are out of medical danger and gaining weight enhances their feelings of control and confidence that the weight they are gaining is being distributed as muscle, not just as fat. A wide range of different methods to achieve weight gain has been explored over the years with the use of supplements combined with muscle-bearing exercise the most widely accepted.

Homework is assigned early on. Following Mary Pipher's practice, which she outlines in her book *Reviving Ophelia*, girls are asked to come up with several qualities they like about themselves and things they don't like. This all can become "food for therapy." The initial sessions are equally divided between talking about their food anxiety and talking about the rest of their lives. Cognitive strategies such as thought interruption and cognitive restructuring are practiced and reinforced. Consciousness-raising is the foundation of our work—from the beginning to the end of psychotherapy.

Consciousness-Raising

In the 1970s the consciousness-raising movement became the largest educational-support movement for women in our history. In a striking parallel, approximately the same number of women then belonged to consciousness-raising groups as are dying each year today of eating disorders. I was part of this political movement, and it was incredibly liberating—a powerful catalyst for women my age to take pride in our sex. We learned how to face life squarely, established goals, began to believe in ourselves and experience great clarity about our true selves. *We became our true selves.* Then feminism died in the 1980s just as it had in the 1920s, and the belief that our problems have both social causes and political solutions died with it. My work with adolescent girls is devoted to bringing to them the same feelings of pride and dignity I experienced in the seventies—a belief that they are essentially worthwhile and interesting human beings who can take control of their eating habits and lives.

Clients are encouraged to watch certain television programs and read different books and magazines in order to determine how images of beauty are used against women. We talk about what they have read and how these magazines and images seem to emphasize women's roles as passive decorative objects. The goal is to help these youngsters break free of the constricting stereotypes of whom they should be. Attempts are made to peel off the beauty mystique of "lookism" with an analysis of how objectification has influenced their body image and eroded their self-esteem. This new consciousness is a process, not a destination. Anorexia is in part a form of self-sacrifice on the altar of ideal beauty, and the unfolding of a new consciousness and feelings of anger directed externally can empower women to think and act differently. We need to encourage our clients to change their values in the same way we were challenged in the sixties and seventies. Linking the political and personal aspects of one's life can be a strong force for healing.

Psychotherapy in Progress

Using one case as an example, the following is an overview of therapeutic techniques used to meet the individual needs of anorexic clients. (I have changed the client's name and other details.) I hope that an account of the process of challenging beliefs and solving problems will illustrate why I am excited and optimistic about the ability of these clients to overcome their disordered eating.

JANE presented herself for therapy for anorexia recently. She is a fifteen-year old high school student who was referred to me by her family friends. Her normal stable weight appears to be a slim 123–126 pounds, and she is tall at 5′8″. She never had any weight problems prior to this episode and has been involved in many sports such as cross-country running and volleyball. About a year ago she became overvigilant about what and how she was eating. She first began to reduce fat and then red meat. A slow weight loss resulted, and as Jane lost weight she became more and more joyless, irritable, and apathetic.

SESSION 1

My first session began with Jane and her mother, Shirley, who was terrified that Jane had damaged her body in significant ways. I reassured her that most of Jane's medical problems were reversible with good nutrition. We spent a good deal of time discussing factual information about how much and what to eat. I pointed out to Jane how her body was, in fact, feeding on itself because she had provided it with no fuel. I discussed the need for her to cut back on aerobic exercises and indicated that weight-bearing exercise would be fine in moderation. I encouraged her family to have a complete medical evaluation done by Jane's PCP. I recommended that they have a consultation with Pat Young, my nutritional consultant, as Jane seemed willing to educate herself about the facts.

I then spent some time talking to Jane alone and weighed her at 116 pounds. Even though her weight loss had been only eight to ten pounds, the impact on her thinking and behavior was profound. On the depression scale Jane indicated she was sad and depressed *a lot* of the time. She was having trouble falling asleep and was waking up too early. She was taking no pleasure in her daily activities and had become less interested in people. She was feeling overwhelmed and fatigued most of the time. I pointed out to her that much of this would disappear as she started to eat better and gain some weight and asked her to keep a food log between now and our next session. I spent time trying to alleviate her fears and promised her she would not gain too much weight and why.

Jane described her childhood and family situation as good and said that she would change nothing about her family life. She said she had a group of about five close girlfriends but no boyfriends. When asked to describe her feelings about herself she said, "Often I feel stressed and angry. I generally like myself, but I'm constantly worrying about being fat. Occasionally I feel like I'm not fun enough or good in sports but not usually." When asked to record what she likes the most about herself, she said, "I make good grades. I have a pretty good reputation." When asked what she wanted to change about herself she indicated, "Not being so worried about fat/calories, to be happier." My impressions of Jane and her family were extremely positive. I liked them all and found Jane to be an articulate, bright, and expressive young woman. All in all it was a good first session.

SESSION 2

I saw Jane again the next day. She expressed many of the classic anorexic fears and distorted irrational beliefs. We went over several of them in detail. In her fear of gaining too much weight, just eating more is terrifying because she has become accustomed to eating nothing. She improved after our session yesterday and actually had steak for dinner. However, she feels guilty. I continue to reinforce the fact that prior to her starvation episode, she was a normal slim person who was quite happy. Since losing weight, she has become obsessed with calories, constantly counting them and always comparing herself to others. She is preoccupied with other girls' bodies—thinking that this one's legs are smaller than hers and so on. Good rapport has been established, and a dialogue developed in which she is listening earnestly and evidencing some trust. We spent the rest of the session troubleshooting specific questions she had about food and exercise.

SESSION 3

A week later I was delighted to see that Jane had gained two pounds. In the interim she had seen her family doctor, her gynecologist, and the nutritionist. Her gynecologist prescribed estrogen and progesterone, and Jane felt the session with Pat, the nutritionist, was extremely helpful. We went over some of the major points—mainly reinforcing the evidence that she can eat a lot more than she believes. She is less phobic about eating and more responsible. However, she felt her parents were "breathing down my back," so we negotiated some new contracts with them to give her more responsibility for her own recovery. I asked her to listen to her father, as she needs to understand his fears just as he needs to understand hers.

I promised Jane that once she starts eating again, her body-image disparagement and distortion will go away. When she said that she had to eat "a lot" over the weekend, I reminded her that she needs to realize that she overestimates what she is eating because her diet has been *minimal amounts of low-calorie food.*

This session I risked allowing Jane to take more control of her eating as an experiment. I do this every chance I can because I want clients to feel they are the "architects," and they can therefore take all the credit. I asked the parents to back off and not constantly watch and comment on what she was eating. This experiment failed abysmally!

SESSION 4
The next session with Jane and her father, Steve, was extremely difficult. When I weighed Jane she weighed 115 1/4 pounds, down from the 118 1/4 pounds of the previous week. She admitted to exercising inappropriately and also owned up to having had a very difficult week. I reinforced her honesty because it took great courage to admit that she had been cheating. Evidently at the beginning of the week she had looked at herself in the mirror and "did not like what she saw." At that point she became very depressed and clearly did whatever she could to undo "the damage." The family became aware of her eating less than the desired amounts, and there were some battles and confrontations. Her father said the younger brother had been acting out as well, so it was really a terrible week. I spent most of the session explaining to Jane the impact of starvation on her body, the reasons for her distorted body image, and the steps that were going to be necessary to get out of danger.

This was a tough-love session, but I also tried to be extremely clear about why she was feeling so bad. We agreed that she needs to stop looking at herself since she does not know what she looks like. Rather, she needs to trust the people who love her to assess how she looks. Also, I do not want her going home after school because that's when she has been exercising and is alone with her thoughts, which are invariably negative and depressing. The family is to help her to have something to do every afternoon until they return home. If she cannot motivate herself to do what she needs to do, then I want to see her, even if it's over the weekend.

SESSION 5

This was a stronger week for Jane; she gained over a pound and felt better. We continued to troubleshoot her "blue moods"—the negative thoughts that precipitate her excessive worrying about what and how she is eating. She began to realize that she has to eat a tremendous amount of food to gain the weight back. We looked at her exercise plan for the week because she was about to start weight training. Since she was going away for the weekend, we discussed whether or not she would exaggerate the amount she ate and come in next week having lost weight. None of us wants to go through that kind of experience again, so the messages were strongly reinforced.

Since Jane is a very capable girl who is strong in most areas of her life, we are working to bring her strengths to bear on this one area where she employs very "undereducated" thinking. We discussed ways that she can start getting control over the negative thinking via cognitive restructuring exercises. For example, I asked her to imagine what I would say whenever she starts struggling with overgeneralizations or all-or-nothing thoughts. At this point she has become fairly well educated about the eating issues and now needs to both listen and talk to herself. We did some role-playing of these thoughts, and I provided the rational response. The types of stops and gos that Jane is experiencing are typical; all in all, she is doing extremely well. She is starting to learn that she is not the best judge of how much she needs to eat. Also, she is starting to realize she is not the bionic woman and that some amount of parental observation and management are necessary.

THESE sessions are good examples of the kind of initial work that is necessary with anorexics. It is grueling and at times frustrating, but it's also very exciting to see these young women learn to control their irrational thoughts.

Who Am I and Who Should I Become?

As work progresses through the middle stages of treatment, less than half of the session is spent on food-related issues. The other half is usually devoted to existential issues, consciousness-raising, and coping strategies.

Almost all clinicians working with and writing about anorexics emphasize the apparent lack of self. Both Hilda Bruch in *Eating Disorders* and Susie Orbach in *Fat is a Feminist Issue* present anorexia as a desperate search for self-worth. Bruch suggests that anorexics lack any reliance on their own thinking: They don't know who they are and what they feel. Orbach suggests the anorexic feels invisible and unknowable to herself and others and that "the making of the individual is the whole raison d'etre of the therapeutic work."

Peggy Claude-Pierre, in her book *The Secret Language of Eating Disorders,* describes two minds at war with each other. The *negative mind* is totally powerful, tyrannical, hypercritical, destructive, and despair confirming, while the *actual mind* is a positive force and consists of normal reactions to everyday events. She too characterizes women with eating disorders as "having no sense of self or identity except for the fulfillment of their extremely subjective perception of other's expectations."

Rather than nonexistent selves, I see girls who were relatively happy until they decided to diet, girls who are talented, insightful, bright, and interesting. However, it is true that along with the significant impact of starvation they have also arrived at an impasse as regards existential issues. They are now at the age where there is more and more pressure to conform to the "false self"—the type of girl society expects. After all, it is precisely the false self—the people pleaser—who is particularly to blame for the fix they are in.

They lack the tools that boys have to distract themselves from pain. They have already developed a ruminative style of thinking that, when combined with the distorted thinking fueled by starvation, causes them to appear much sicker than they really are.

In my work therapy is presented as an exciting journey with the destination of becoming real—an opportunity to develop character and new identities. I agree with Orbach and Pipher that therapy can provide a milieu in which women can unfold and discover their true selves. This type of awakening always provides the most exciting moments in therapy. It is the "Aha!" moments—those lightbulbs going off—that warm my heart as girls start to develop insights and become energized to take action and change their lives.

Changing Values

My aim is to combine consciousness-raising with cognitive therapy in a process of cognitive restructuring to change not only thinking but entrenched stereotyped values as well. The different ways boys and girls handle pain is discussed along with the differences researchers have found in styles of thinking. The goal is to inspire and excite them about their ability to change, grow, and develop dignity. They are educated about their poor coping strategies, shown how they have been brainwashed, and challenged to start questioning the unfairness of their unequal relationships. Why should they think more about their boyfriends than their boyfriends think about them? Why should their boyfriends spend their time involved in pursuing instrumental skills and developing new identities while they spend much of their time with girlfriends shopping, doing nails—obsessed with their looks. They agree that boys almost never give up any of their identities, including hanging out with their boyfriends, to be with them.

Therapy is a constant process of questioning values and presenting alternatives. The young women I see are confronted about how their thinking and activities limit their freedom, sap their energy, and consume valuable time—time that could be better spent enhancing existing identities and/or developing new ones. Their lives could be more self-fulfilling, more fun. These "male or female" characteristics are not *genetic*. They are learned and can be un-learned. Girls need to believe that they have the capacity to develop new skills and become competent in them.

Changing Thinking

The different forms of twisted thinking that cognitive therapist David Burns has identified in his book *Feeling Good* are "food for therapy." They include: all-or-nothing thinking, overgeneraliza-tion, mental filter, discounting the positive, jumping to conclu-sions, magnification/minimization, emotional reasoning, "should" statements, labeling, and personalization. Clients make a list of these ten forms of twisted thinking and then write down every time they become depressed or anxious during the week. For homework, they are asked to engage in a three-step process. First they must ask themselves: "What am I telling myself?"—identify the depressed or anxious automatic thought. Second, they are to identify which form or forms of twisted thinking they are em-ploying. The third step is to verbalize a more rational and con-structive self-statement.

I give the following example: "Yesterday my best friend, Mary, walked right by me at the mall without speaking. My automatic re-action is to become very depressed and think, What have I done? Why is Mary angry with me? I must have done something to her." (These are the types of statements that lead to depression or anxi-ety. Many girls spend hours obsessing about similar events, tor-turing themselves needlessly.) Now let's go to the second step and identify the irrational beliefs: "I am jumping to conclusions based on limited information as well as personalizing the event; i.e., "It's all my fault." The third step involves coming up with a more ra-tional explanation: "Oh, well, I guess she didn't see me, and I'll have to ask her about this when I see her at school. Let go of it, and don't let this ruin your day."

Clients keep a journal, and we work on these times of depression and anxiety by analyzing and restructuring the irrational assumptions until the new rational thoughts become the new habit that begins to eliminate the old style of needless rumination and torture. When we look at the *belief* of not hurting his or her feelings, the point is made how this is an excuse to hide behind a lack of courage and how they are making an insulting assumption that the other person is weak and incapable of handling feedback. They examine their own beliefs about whether or not they would rather receive direct and honest feedback than confusing "mixed messages." (They would!) They work on how they can give feedback in a gentle manner, and they learn not to confuse assertiveness with aggression.

Role-playing helps them feel comfortable expressing their feelings honestly. "Initiating, initiating, initiating" is a constant theme. Girls too often passively wait for things to happen instead of creating their own settings. Cognitive work always admonishes them to look rationally at the worst thing that could happen if they take risks and to rationally determine if it is catastrophic or uncomfortable. Ninety-nine percent of the time it is uncomfortable. The focus is on problem-solving in a solution-based manner. Our motto becomes, "If it's hard—do it, and if you don't want to do it—do it." Another female ritual that subtracts from women, crying, is targeted. Growing up as girls we were encouraged to cry: "You will feel better if you let it all out." I disagree. I find that girls cry instead of talk and act. Boys are told to get a grip on themselves. Clients are asked to find the words to express their pain instead of crying. Eventually they are able to attenuate this form of helplessness and hopelessness admirably while learning to communicate their needs. They are challenged to consider why boys handle criticism better. How can they learn to be as strong?

Compliments and Strokes

In role-playing, clients practice accepting criticism and receiving compliments with grace. Girls are horrible at accepting compliments. The famous psychoanalyst Alfred Adler identified the importance of our social world as a source of positive reinforcement and urged his clients to elicit strokes, receive them graciously, and give them to others regularly.

A particular problem for women is that they often receive strokes for engaging in activities they don't value—for example, cleaning the house so nicely. Someone saying: "I'm proud of the way you handled that obnoxious salesman—*you were outstanding!*" is a different story. Most of us—men and women—would welcome this feedback. However, in order to elicit it, we have to take risks and become involved socially. I encourage clients to "dream"—dream of an activity or event they could participate in that would make them feel good about themselves, resulting in strokes that would be truly meaningful. Self-respect and confidence are derived from triumphing over obstacles. They also need to reach inside and develop the ability to stroke themselves more instead of always looking for outside validation from others.

We work on how girls too automatically deflect compliments and why refusing to accept them with grace subtracts from them and is a slap in the face to the person who handed them this gift—the compliment. It also reveals their poor self-esteem and is often so annoying that it effectively eliminates potential sources of strokes. The problem is that most of us do not receive strokes regularly, so if we deflect the few we do get, we will maintain our poor self-image and continue to feel bad. Therefore, we need to accept strokes with grace and savor them over and over.

We also work on *giving* strokes. Sometimes the "false self"—the people pleaser—is insincere in stroking others. Girls are given all kinds of messages telling them to be nice, considerate, and "appropriate." This works against acting without fear. To speak authentically demands courage and risk taking.

Anger

The most difficult emotion for clients to express genuinely is anger. Anger is not a characteristic of the people pleaser. As Sanford and Donovan wrote in *Women and Self-Esteem* (1985), "An angry woman is despised as a bitch or put down as maladjusted or sexually unsatisfied." Thus there is anxiety and confusion about expressing anger. We identify anger as "depression turned inward or stuffed feelings" leading to "learned helplessness." It is not surprising that another syndrome—that of self-injury—also called self-mutilation—has been connected to pushing down feelings of anger. In an article in *Counseling Today* (March 1999), David Kaplan, the president of the International Association of Marriage and Family Counselors, states: "We teach women to turn anger in on themselves, and we teach men to turn anger outward—boys drive 90 miles an hour or fight, women blame themselves. That's why there are so many more eating disorders in women as compared to men."

I believe that Kaplan is entirely right, and expressing anger appropriately is a major focus in therapy. Role-playing and assertiveness training are enormously useful as clients learn acceptable ways of expressing feelings and discover that one of their most important challenges is to constructively express angry feelings to someone without guilt or the excuse of not wanting to hurt his/her feelings.

Cognitive therapy and consciousness-raising work together to help clients spend less time denying or suppressing their feelings. With practice, the majority begin to feel a sense of pride and dignity about their ability to be authentic, and once they do, it becomes extremely difficult to return to being a passive, nonassertive people pleaser.

Overcoming Body Hatred and Self-Neglect

Another difficult task is to help clients change their body dissatisfaction and develop more realistic and kinder ways of evaluating themselves. Within our sessions we discuss the ways our culture teaches us to hate our bodies and how we become our own worst enemies and critics. We talk about ridiculous ideals and the way body hatred saps our energy, time, and spirit. We analyze the different ways boys and girls feel about their bodies, and we look for reasons why. Why should girls waste their time obsessing when they can be striving for excellence in arenas that allow a triumph of their intellect, spirit, and sense of who they are? In place of worrying about their bodies, can they experience pleasure and relaxation? This is another major problem. Everything is work and no play, and clients have difficulty engaging in refueling and pleasurable "selfish" activities. Reverse brainwashing is obviously necessary.

I remember this liberating insight in therapy. A therapist asked me: "What do you do for fun?" I was a wife and mother in the sixties, so of course I responded, "I don't do anything for fun." He questioned, "Why?" Like many of my clients today, it had never occurred to me that it was all right for me to engage in fun activities—that was "frivolous." Since I couldn't come up with anything, the therapist told me to "dream." I realized that I had always fantasized about riding horses, skiing, and engaging in photography. The therapist then told me to find out about resources for all these activities in the community before our next session. In essence, he gave me permission to challenge my thinking. After all, why was it OK for my husband to engage in several of his hobbies and interests when my life was spent as a caretaker? I found out there was a Cornell horseback riding class, a six-week ski lesson package for Cornell staff, and a photography course being offered at a different college. In essence, that moment was the beginning of an avocational life. I began to participate in all three of these interests, and thirty years later they are major identities as well as coping strategies for me.

Overwhelmingly, anorexic girls are overachievers, extremely perfectionistic and hardworking. Helping them to engage in fun activities without feeling guilty may be one of the most important coping strategies we can teach them along with adaptive mood-management techniques.

Relationships with Boys

Boys, relationships, and the whole concept of rejection are explored through consciousness-raising. Girls are asked to consider the following: "Let's pretend that you have a computer that can be wired to your boyfriend's thoughts and your thoughts. Every time he thinks about you, the computer goes *blip,* and every time you think about him, it will go *blip.* At the end of the week we will pull the tapes out and compare them. What will we find?" This question is usually enough in itself to start eliciting knowing laughter from my clients. But why should they think more about boys than boys think about them?

Nolen-Hoeksema and colleagues (1993, 1998) asked male and female college students to record their experiences of depressed moods and what they did in response to these moods each day for a month. The women were significantly more likely than men to report engaging in ruminative, self-focused responses to their depressed moods, such as thinking about how tired and alone they felt. We examine these studies in order to consider alternatives and to realize that the women are behaviorally and emotionally impoverished and need to develop new survival skills. Eventually they get mad, and getting mad is a powerful facilitator for change.

The Middle to the Beginning

It is virtually impossible to do time-limited psychotherapy with anorexics; the length of time needed varies enormously. As we have seen from Jane's case, therapy is often a series of successes, followed by failures, followed by more successes, more failures, and so on. I usually see anorexics for six months to two years. I have learned by trial and error that therapy should not be terminated until the girl has achieved her stable specific weight. In my experience, the women who become chronic and continue to have episodes of anorexia are those who achieved only a suboptimal weight even though they were considered to be no longer anorexic. Their bodies are still so vulnerable to sickness and stress that typically a crisis or illness can result in a ten-pound weight loss. At this point these women usually come back in for booster sessions, but most of the problem still seems to be trying to maintain a biologically impossible ideal. In addition, in their state of semistarvation they will continue to evidence pessimistic anorexic thinking patterns. (As we will see later, the need for long-term treatment of one to two years for the anorexic need not become a battle with managed care companies if treatment goals are logically specified step by step.)

In the middle stages of therapy it is possible to see the clients at longer intervals. Two weeks between sessions gives them a lot more to practice, experience, and talk about in the session. By the middle of therapy the client has typically become weight restored and is fully engaged in a program of nutritional rehabilitation. Now is the time to work on maintaining the weight and transforming all of the intellectual insights into genuine risk taking and success— engaging in activities to lift their moods instead of focusing on their feelings when they are down, decatastrophizing rejection, speaking up, acting up, saying no.

When women begin to like what they are doing, they begin to like themselves. Soon they become prouder of handling a difficult situation well than losing a few pounds. Neophyte therapists believe they "cure" people. After practicing psychotherapy for twenty-five years I have discovered this to be wrong. *Clients cure themselves!* The *easy* part is our session; the *hard* part is what they do when they leave our offices. The reason I have engaged in this work is I love watching people grow. I am glad to be a small part of the process, but the truth is our clients need to take most of the responsibility for their own personal triumphs in overcoming their eating disorders.

11 .

Surviving Managed Care

In 1991 Bill and I had a thriving practice in both our Radford and Roanoke, Virginia, offices. We were well-known and respected and worked closely with many physicians, colleges, and schools. Our referrals came from everywhere. Bill was trained as a child psychologist and was an exceptionally good one. He developed contracts with many of the school systems and provided psychological assessments for children referred to him. I continued to specialize in the treatment of eating disorders but also began to branch out, treating other women's issues as well. I became interested in the problems of infertility, postpartum depression, and high-risk pregnancies after one of my daughters had these problems. Several of the gynecologists began to refer clients to me. After surviving breast cancer, I began to treat this population as well. Bill and I were enjoying our work and leisure time greatly. In fact, we were slowly starting to back off from work and thinking ahead to retirement.

Then in the fall of 1991 our state's largest health insurer merged with a huge managed-care company. Suddenly our secure, safe practice was being threatened. We were told in effect that we had to join up or get out. If we had not joined, we would have had to rely on clients who could afford to pay the bills themselves. But clients with indemnity insurance were the core of my practice, and at this stage of my career it was unrealistic to run a successful practice built on private-pay clients. The years we had devoted to our practice, our expertise, our good reputation, didn't seem to matter.

Rather, we were given very explicit rules about how to conduct therapy and also how to document what we were doing. They expected me to treat anorexics in six sessions or less. Like many clinicians, I was finding my ability to control my practice and my feelings of competence ebbing away. As colleague Dr. Dana C. Ackley in *Breaking Free of Managed Care* (1997) put it: "If they could get the results they claimed in so few sessions, what was wrong with me?" I had always adhered to a short-term treatment plan, and in fact sometimes I was able to end treatment after six sessions. But the protocol I had been given looked nothing like how I practiced psychotherapy. They wanted me to discuss my client's problems in terms of disease categories and fill out outpatient treatment reports (OTRs) and engage in phone utilization reviews after every few sessions.

Next, we learned that several other managed-care companies were taking over businesses in the area. Now the issue was to get on their provider lists; some were already shutting out providers, having found therapists who were willing to work for lower pay, longer hours, and less autonomy. Our experience with this first HMO turned out to be a worst-case scenario. (The state fired them after four years, but unfortunately there are still too many like them.) My reputation did help me to get on most provider panels. The real problems began to occur when I filled out OTRs requesting additional sessions. The first time I submitted a treatment plan, it came back with the words NEED SPECIFICS, NEED SPECIFICS all over it. This is the original OTR I submitted:

O.T.R.

PRESENTING PROBLEM *(include precipitating stressors, onset, duration, current symptoms, impact on daily functioning)*: Anorexia Nervosa—(cyclical) since age 11. Weight varies from 95–130, presently Mary is 95. No purging other than compulsive and unrelenting exercise. Eats nothing for weeks at a time whenever environmental problems occur; i.e., stress related to schoolwork, relationships with men, etc. History of sexual abuse.

DIAGNOSIS: *Axis I—Anorexia Nervosa   II—Post Traumatic Stress Syndrome related to sexual abuse   III   IV   V

MEDICAL HISTORY/MEDICATION: History of fainting, fatigue, electrolyte disturbances related to starving.

TREATMENT HISTORY: Mary has sought therapy 2Xs in the last few years. Both experiences were not helpful, with Mary quitting after a few sessions. She maintains that therapists were not knowledgeable about eating disorders and did not provide insight, direction, or strategies.

PROBLEMS TO BE ADDRESSED *(Include Symptoms):* Eliminate starving and compulsive exercise and replace with nutritional rehabilitation. Normalize eating and body image disturbance. Provide reassurance and education re how much she can eat, what to eat, how much to exercise, etc. Process sexual abuse issues. Mary has never discussed or worked on these problems previously.

GOALS *(In Behavioral Terms):* See initial progress note. 1. Weight restoration (needs to gain 10 pounds) and nutritional rehabilitation; 2. Resolve sexual abuse issues; 3. Enhance and sophisticate coping strategies so that starving will no longer be an automatic response when life becomes difficult; 4) Initiate social life and avocational interests.

METHODOLOGY: Use cognitive behavioral tools, behavioral modification, and strategies delineated in *Bulimarexia: Binge/Purge Cycle*—2nd ed. 1987, W. W. Norton. We will attempt to alter the above maladaptive behaviors as well as providing support and psychotherapy re: the sexual abuse.

DATE OF FIRST SERVICE: _____

TOTAL NUMBER OF SESSIONS DELIVERED AS OF THIS REQUEST: 8 _____

---

*Axes are different domains of information that help the clinician plan treatment and predict outcome. There are five axes included in the DSM IV (American Psychiatric Association: Diagnostic and Statistical Manual of Mental Disorders). The five axes are:

Axis I	Clinical Disorders
Axis II	Personality Disorders/Mental Retardation
Axis III	General Medical Conditions
Axis IV	Psychosocial and Environmental Problems
Axis V	Global Assessment of Functioning (GAF)

ADDITIONAL SESSIONS REQUESTED: 24 TYPE: Individual: 12
FAMILY:____ GROUP: 12 if Mary is able to secure transportation to
Roanoke
FREQUENCY: 1x per week ESTIMATED ADDITIONAL # OF SESSIONS
TO COMPLETE TREATMENT: 20 Group; 20 Individual

In answer to SPECIFICS, I wrote the following letter:

Dear—

I am writing to address the issues you posed in your correspondence
dated December 30, 1993. Mary is 5′2″ tall and weighs approximately 95
pounds. The diagnosis for Mary is as follows:

AXIS I: Anorexia Nervosa (307.10) and Post-Traumatic Stress Syndrome
Related to Sexual Abuse (309.81)
AXIS II: No diagnosis
AXIS III: Serious medical implications secondary to starving and anorexia
nervosa; i.e., chronic fatigue and electrolyte disturbances.
AXIS IV: Psychosocial stressors. Living circumstances: move from New
York to Virginia. Interpersonal—breakup of a long-term relationship
with a man. Post-traumatic stress related to childhood sexual abuse; i.e.,
night terrors, panic attacks, etc. Severity: 4—moderate.
AXIS V: Current GAF: 56/Highest GAF past year: 45

Mary has been referred to Dr. Jones. He has medically managed eating-
disordered students at Virginia State College for several years and we
work as a team. Mary will see him for the appropriate medical evaluation
and tests once she resumes classes after January 17. She may or may not
require medication if her electrolytes are deficient and/or Dr. Jones may
recommend *inpatient hospitalization* in an eating-disorder program if
there is a medical necessity to do so. My belief is the only "medicine" she
requires is *food*. Presently, she does not require antidepressant therapy
because she is motivated and willing to work on her problems.

GOALS *(specifics):* Cognitive restructuring, targeting body image disturbance, misperception, and disparagement; phobic reactions to
eating, feeling full, and an assortment of other classic anorexic beliefs such as:

1. I have a disease, a mental illness;
2. I have been anorexic for years, therefore it will take years to recover;
3. Unless I understand *why* I starve, I'll never be able to recover; and
4. Starving and excessive exercise are the best weight control methods.

Begin to process sexual abuse issues *only after* there is some normalization of eating.

Have Mary begin involvement in eating-disorders group I am starting in February for college women.

METHODOLOGY *(further specifics):* Help Mary face anxiety and situations associated with eating; e.g., eating in public via examinations of thoughts and personal meanings underlying anxiety behavior such as "Everyone will think I'm a pig," "Everyone will be watching me eat," "If I start eating, I won't be able to stop," etc. We will attempt to eliminate these catastrophic thoughts of gloom associated with these events, and I will have Mary keep a log of dysfunctional thoughts associated with anxiety as well as a food and mood diary. Between sessions I will have Mary take specific risks such as eating with a friend who understands her problem, etc. Also, I have already submitted a very detailed chapter I have written, delineating many other strategies I have devised that have helped hundreds of anorexics/bulimics in their recovery. Please refer to this chapter for more specific information.

I hope this information will clear up any problems you have with authorizing sessions for Mary. We have established good rapport and work well together. Please advise me as soon as possible of your decision as I am seeing Mary weekly and need to advise her parents of any problems having insurance cover these sessions. I saw Mary on _____, and today _____, without having a decision from you on authorizations. Your prompt attention to this matter is greatly appreciated.

Sincerely,
Marlene Boskind-White, Ph.D., L.P.C., L.M.F.T.

All of this documentation was ignored, and I received another denial that led to a second lengthy letter expressing my confusion and dismay. I begged for more sessions with Mary, carefully addressing her needs and the critical nature of our work together. Eventually I received authorization for additional sessions; however, my credentials and years of experience seemed meaningless to these people: *They* knew how to treat women with eating disorders, and *I* didn't. By 1995 I was completely out of control and didn't give a damn. I was certain I was going to be bounced off the provider panel and had reached the point where I hardly cared.

Although I usually won on appeal, I spent hours of unreimbursed time providing documentation that the company did not even seem to read. Although angry, I felt I had to advocate for my clients no matter what, so I saw no other choice. Over the next three years things got worse.

Fortunately, after this company left the state I found other MOs to be reasonable and professional. I was able to interact with case managers in an atmosphere of mutual respect and partnership. For example, the following letter led to sessions being approved after a denial without any problems whatsoever.

Dear _____:

This letter is an attempt to reverse a decision your company has made in disallowing Nancy additional psychotherapy sessions. My treatment of Nancy for anorexia nervosa has been stimulating, often frustrating, but also extremely rewarding. A total cure has not been achieved completely, but Nancy has evidenced adequate daily functioning and has made some significant psychological growth. She still suffers from occasional severe depressive episodes and anxiety.

Over the last year our strong therapeutic alliance has allowed very productive work to occur in *brief* individual sessions occurring at long intervals; i.e., one half hour individual session per month. Also, Nancy's involvement in her group (she usually attends every other week) for recovering eating-disordered clients has helped enormously in her search for autonomy and a self-directed identity. In this setting of new intimate interpersonal relationships, what she has to say is listened to and made the focus of exploration and respect. She has desperately needed a sense of connectedness to peers, and the group allows her a forum for expressing her feelings about her father's alcoholism and her mother's overbearing, intrusive involvement in her life. Thus, brief sessions have been quite successful in preventing relapse.

The treatment for anorexia nervosa is broadly divided into two phases:

initial weight restoration—usually conducted within an inpatient set-ting—and psychotherapy aimed at preventing relapse. We were very for-tunate indeed that the weight restoration aspect of treatment occurred on an outpatient basis with a minimum of subterfuge and resistance. Thus inpatient hospitalization was successfully averted. Since fully 30 percent of anorexics relapse, obviously a major task has been to keep a lapse from becoming a relapse or a collapse. Recently Nancy's weight loss of eight pounds was nipped in the bud and restored quickly. She continues to need help in improving her self-esteem. Her sense of self-worth is still rigidly tied to external frames of reference, and she still experiences her-self as ineffective, incompetent, and vulnerable to external control—es-pecially when she has to deal with any type of crisis, disappointment, or rejection. Nancy's automatic response under these circumstances is still to resort to old strategies like starvation. Thus an essential part of our work together has been the gradual modification of her cognitive appraisal sys-tems and underlying assumptions related to her self-esteem. This has been accomplished by consistent cognitive behavioral interventions. For example, Nancy's sense of self-worth is too exclusively tied to acceptance from others, and so nonacceptance often produces anxiety and depression and starvation. Much of my work lies in guiding this patient in ques-tioning how she evaluates herself. Nancy evaluates others' worth by the same inflexible criteria that she uses for herself. These brief sessions always have great impact and lead to significant changes in Nancy's behaviors and attitudes.

In summary, I hope you will support what I consider very reasonable and much needed brief, occasional individual and group therapy ses-sions. Nancy and her mother both feel extremely anxious about your de-nial of further benefits in this regard, and I hope this letter will help you reconsider and respect the value of our request.

Sincerely,
Marlene Boskind-White, Ph.D., L.P.C., L.M.F.T.

Whether we like it or not, managed care is here to stay. It was born in the early 1980s after health-care costs had doubled in a decade and the government wanted to begin shifting costs from the public to the private sector. While it has become successful in con-trolling soaring costs, it has also taken health-care decisions out of the hands of clients and their doctors. Case managers hired by insurers now make these decisions for us. Yet what form managed care will take in the future is far from clear.

The late 1990s have seen an unprecedented act of rebellion on the part of physicians, who feel managed care has robbed them of autonomy, quality of care, income, time, prestige, and even self-respect. Many are dropping out of health maintenance organization contracts, filing lawsuits, seeking redress in their professional organizations, and even considering unions that are now competing to capitalize on physicians' frustrations. Others are retiring early or moving to new areas not overtaken by managed-care organizations (MCOs). Hundreds of physicians en masse have refused contracts in California, Texas, Florida, Georgia, and Colorado.

Managed care presents particular problems for mental health practitioners. Fees have been slashed and will continue to fall as benefits are being squeezed. Furthermore, graduate schools are turning out large numbers of social workers, counselors, and clinical psychologists. New providers also undercut the market in order to be included on panels.

Recently the HMO Magellan "amended" rates for psychologists by 30 percent, from $72.00 to $50.00 in an outpatient session. Master-level clinicians were reduced 28 percent, from $63.00 to $45.00. Some wonder if this is not just another ploy to get providers to drop out since Magellan has more network behavioral health providers than they need.

Another trend ahead is integration of primary and behavioral health care, seen by some as inevitable. Unless we are able to run a 100 percent private-pay practice with clients who can afford to stay in therapy as long as they want, the integration trend will effect us. Otherwise, if we want to remain in practice, we will need to cultivate more relationships with physicians. GPs are moving into the driver's seat and landing jobs as gatekeepers for most types of health care organizations.

Since MCOs involve direct clinical management, confidentiality is a serious issue as well. Some MCOs now want total access to network providers' *financial records,* not simply clinical information.

The issue grows as an increasing number of small groups and sole practices align with group practices—at least on a part-time basis. Around-the-clock service is now a must for provider groups working with managed care and Employee Assistance programs (EAP).

The bottom line is this: Therapists who want to work outside managed care have to market and promote their practices.

Working with Managed Care

As a therapist treating eating disorders and assisting clients to access their health insurance benefits, I face many dilemmas and obstacles. On the one hand managed care has eliminated some of the abuses I found offensive and frightening in the eighties. The inpatient eating-disorder programs that were marketing their services in aggressive and outrageous ways have largely disappeared. However, with the elimination of inpatient programs there are fewer resources for the chronic anorexic who may be in a life-threatening situation.

Before managed care, third parties did not focus as much on pathology. Now, in order to fill out OTRs and justify our sessions to reviewers, we much consistently document symptoms. In order for my clients to utilize insurance, I must diagnose them with a mental illness. Since I believe eating disorders are habits that are learned and can be unlearned, I am already faced with a catch-22. Rather than being able to focus on strengths and changing values, I am now required to describe my work in ways I find offensive: disease categories.

The more serious the symptoms, the greater the likelihood that we will win reimbursement. However, if the client appears *too chronic,* the MCO might use that as an excuse to terminate our work together. Everything that is harmful about the individual's pathology model in eating disorders is reinforced in our contracts with MCOs. Clients and their therapists are forced to focus on their weaknesses and assign labels in order to get reimbursed.

Dana C. Ackley (1997) discusses the dangers of this model:

"Suggesting to people that they are sick, helpless, or not responsible, an inherent component in the medical model, promotes failure and dependency. Too often people become their diagnosis."

Another ethical dilemma is the obvious loss of privacy as a result of the constant documentation that is now required. It is all too easy for medical secrets to find their way out of a doctor's files. Clients who were hospitalized for anorexia in adolescence may find themselves unable to get into the college of their choice, denied employment, or unable to purchase insurance. Only recently has the Federal Trade Commission begun requiring companies to tell consumers when information about their prior medical history has adversely affected them. Most of the time we have no idea what happens to the information we submit when clients sign release forms for giving information to managed care. Serious legal implications are raised for the providers too when clients damaged by a release of this information might hold them responsible.

For the time being, most of us have had to embrace a quiet resignation to what has happened to our practices and the way we conduct them. The growth phase for managed behavioral health care seems to be slowing down with most of the mergers now completed. Today there are only a handful of MCOs, which has caused them to pay a heavy price—many are now posting losses. Most of us will have to wait for mental health parity laws as well as federal legislation. These "fairness bills" are pending in several states; in Virginia, managed care is the focus of a 1999 general assembly currently under way. A "patient's bill of rights" includes fourteen provisions ranging from changing health-plan liability to allowing any specialist to become a primary-care provider as well as sweeping alterations in provider network laws. Until then, proactive independence in our profession will take a backseat to a financially dependent position.

Not only are MCOs here to stay, they do not need us as providers! They typically have far more providers than they want, so the key is to develop a collaborative relationship built upon mutual respect that does not compromise integrity. The following are some suggestions and coping skills I've developed in dealing with managed care. Over the years many have been discussed in detail in a very helpful practice resource for behavioral health providers called *Psychotherapy Finances.*

Contracts with HMOs

Read contracts carefully before signing, ask questions about confusing areas, and let a lawyer read the contract and advise you. Know your obligations and the limitations that may be imposed, and don't sign up with companies that provide little or no information about themselves. Remember that contracts are not set in stone and can be negotiated and altered.

Writing Managed Care–Friendly Treatment Plans

1. Delineate your proposed treatment in a defined time-limited manner. A treatment plan must be structured and goal focused. It must provide a full profile of the client outlining the nature of the crisis and the purpose of treatment. Goals must be stated in measurable behavioral terms indicating specific progress to be made within given time periods. The course of treatment should be aimed at symptom reduction within a reasonable number of sessions. (Don't ask for too much at one time even if the client is in dire need; otherwise, the MCO will believe you want to keep the client in treatment forever.) OTRs should be submitted on time and completely filled out according to the MCO's criteria.
2. The time requested for the sessions should be appropriate for the diagnosis.
3. A methodology for the treatment and criteria that underline the specific diagnosis must be spelled out.
4. To show you can facilitate early discharge, provide well-designed plans for utilizing adjunctive/collateral services such as Alcoholic Anonymous, groups for survivors of sexual abuse, cancer support groups, bereavement groups, and so on. This

shows the MCO that you are aware of and willing to refer clients to other levels of care and resources that complement and reinforce treatment goals.

5. If you plan to recommend hospitalization or psychiatric evaluation, have documentation that strongly justifies this plan.
6. Link clinical improvement to specific interventions, and detail a predischarge level of progress.
7. Know limits and structures of specific benefits. Some may only be three sessions and others twenty.
8. Make the role of other professionals essential to the outcome of this case, such as psychiatrists for management of any medications and nutritionists for nutritional rehabilitation.
9. Understand, identify, and plan how to handle potential crisis situations.
10. Keep copies of everything. Many times insurers say plans have not been received or they will be received and then lost.
11. Mail rather than fax reports, or do both simultaneously.
12. If there are billing problems, keep cool; don't bill clients or have them call the company. This always backfires.

The following are a few sample outpatient treatment reports for eating-disordered clients. The first is for an anorexic.

Risk History

Explain any significant history of suicidal, homicidal, impulse control, medical, or substance-abuse behavior that may affect client's level of risk or impairment to functioning:

Client has been hospitalized as an inpatient on two occasions for severe starvation related to anorexia nervosa. On both occasions the client's weight dropped significantly, from 120 to 85 pounds (the first hospitalization) and to 100 pounds (the second). Client has attended on-campus group for eating disorders but does not want to return because group is composed of overweight women she cannot identify with.

[*Note:* Telling the MCO that support services were recommended and refused by the client and why underlines the fact that you are not fostering dependency and that discharge and relapse prevention are being considered at all times. The *whole person* is being assessed not just the dynamics occurring in the therapy session.]

Functional Impairments

Explain how the client's symptoms impair functioning in each area below, or place client at risk. Severity rating: 1=mild; 2=moderate; 3=severe

AREA	SEVERITY	DESCRIPTION
Job/School	*3*	*Starvation has contributed to great difficulties in concentration. Client has missed several classes and may need to leave the university if weight restoration and nutritional rehabilitation do not occur immediately.*
Relationship/ Family	*2*	*Little contact with family. Many relationships with peers have ended because of eating disorder. Friends feel she has "too many problems."*

Current Medication

X NONE   PSYCHIATRIC   MEDICAL   NO INFORMATION
PRESCRIBED BY: *X* PSYCHIATRIST   OTHER PHYSICIAN
SPECIFY *(include dosage, frequency and compliance):* Client was withdrawn from Prozac because of side effects related to agitation and restlessness. Psychiatrist is also concerned about utilizing medication when client's medical condition is so precarious.

[NOTE: The MCO needs to know why the client is not on medication. Telling them up front like this reduces the probability of further hassles and illustrates that a psychiatrist has been consulted. In terms of the risk history, any time you can show risk, you are building more of a case for medical necessity.]

Diagnosis

*Axis I—Primary: 307.1 Anorexia Nervosa   Secondary: None
*Axis II: None

*Axis III: Myriad medical problems associated with starvation
*Axis IV (identify stressors): Client has been missing classes and is fearful of flunking out of school.
*Axis V: (GAF) Current 65 Highest in last 12 months: 60

Treatment Goals

Progress rating scale: N=new goal; 1=much worse; 2=somewhat worse; 3=no change; 4=slight improvement; 5=great improvement; R=resolved

Measurable Behavioral Goals

1. Stabilize medical condition via weight restoration and nutritional rehabilitation. Client needs to gain 10 pounds. Weight is presently 100 pounds. Height is 5′2″. Weight gain should be in increments of 1/2–1 pound per week.
2. Restructure distorted thoughts, beliefs, and values that contribute to eating disorder.
3. Maintain mood stability as evidenced by self-report and weight gain.

Methods for Achieving Goal

1. Utilize psychoeducational information about the impact of starvation, and connect it to the client's apathy, irritability, and problems in concentration.
   PROGRESS (since last report) 4
   TARGET DATE TO RESOLVE THIS GOAL: Ongoing—will need to gain 10 pounds, maintain weight, and not settle for suboptimal weight. Will need booster sessions for some time.
2. Use of cognitive restructuring to address irrational beliefs about how to eat, what to eat, how much to exercise, fears of becoming fat, and unacceptable feelings of fullness.
   PROGRESS (since last report) 5
   TARGET DATE TO RESOLVE THIS GOAL: Ongoing. There will be major improvements in thinking and body image once nutritional rehabilitation is under way.
3. Mood management and coping skills. Assertiveness to help clients express feelings, reality therapy to help client understand parent's panic about the serious implications of her starvation.
   PROGRESS (SINCE LAST REPORT) 4

TARGET DATES TO RESOLVE GOALS: 3–6 months (for above goals as well).

[Note that treatment goals are described in concrete behavioral goals and interventions. The target date does not specify time that is too far away in the future. However, the MCO needs to be aware of the fact that anorexia is a serious, life-threatening disorder that does not lend itself to a short-term psychotherapy model.]

The next is a sample of a different type of treatment plan for bulimarexia, the binge/purge cycle.

PRESENTING PROBLEMS
1. Severe binge/purge cycle 3X per day for 4 years.
2. Severe self-disparagement and distorted body image.
3. Irrational fear of becoming overweight.
4. Depressed, can't concentrate, agitated with some suicidal ideation. Denies intent.

PRIOR INPATIENT AND/OR OUTPATIENT MH/SA TREATMENT. (LIST NAMES OF PROVIDERS, REASONS FOR TREATMENT.)

DESCRIBE CURRENT FUNCTIONAL IMPAIRMENT NOTING SPECIFIC BEHAVIORS, EMOTIONS, AND THOUGHT PROCESSES. *Include severity, frequency and situational factors. Be specific.* Client has been stealing roommate's food when bingeing and then goes days without eating. Recently she feels hopeless and helpless about ever overcoming her problem. She is not sleeping well, is extremely depressed, and is highly anxious.

SPECIAL CONCERNS Client needs to be monitored by PCP to make sure outpatient psychotherapy is appropriate and hospitalization not necessary.

GOALS
1. Attenuate and ultimately eliminate severe cycle of bingeing and purging.
2. Restore normal eating patterns, body weight, and realistic perceptions of body size.
3. Restructure distorted thoughts that maintain binge/purge cycle; e.g., "Once I start eating, I can't stop," and develop coping strategies for stressful situations so that bingeing is not a number-one response in the hierarchy.

For telephone utilization reviews, have all of your ducks lined up before you speak to a case manager. Have the session dates and the DSM codes with GAF ready before you call, and be prepared to offer brief and to the point summaries. Make sure you provide accurate data such as spelling of client's name and the correct Social Security number.

In filling out OTRs, type them or write very neatly. Be thorough, but don't go into great detail. (Case managers complain that either the therapist is not specific enough or tells too much.)

Spell out the diagnosis as well as the diagnostic code. Don't make the case manager figure out what you mean so that they have to refer to the DSM. Become familiar with each company's procedures. Whenever possible I talk to the case managers myself, even if a secretary could have performed the same function. Providers who have the highest degree of success with managed care are the ones who adopt a friendly system for following up and following through with their contacts. Many therapists fail to do this once they get on the panel. My last strategy for decreasing the likelihood that I will be targeted by MCOs for disinfranchisement is to always be prepared to see a client they ask me to see as soon as possible.

Everywhere we turn in the field the term "marketing" appears. The idea that psychotherapy and marketing go together is still something I struggle with and find offensive. However, there are ways to build our practices and make our services known without compromising integrity.

Strategies for Eating-Disorder Specialists

The following are some of the strategies eating disorder specialists have found helpful:

1. Conduct workshops, seminars and presentations. I am always available for free lectures. I feel those of us who make our living treating eating disorders have a responsibility to educate the public about prevention. Recently, a half-hour talk to a local pri-

vate high school led to newspaper articles as well as a local news feature shown on two different television stations. As a result, I received an enormous response from people who saw the TV programs.

2. Group therapy for eating disorders has always been an adjunct to my individual work, and in the increasingly competitive market of managed care, effective group therapy may soon be a requirement for inclusion on most managed-care panels. Some predict that in a few years groups will comprise somewhere between a third to half of all treatments. Managed care clearly likes group therapy, and they are committed to using it more and more. However, not just anyone can do a group, and MCOs are looking for competent clinicians who have documented training and experience in running groups for eating disorders.

A group-therapy program should be presented as following a cognitive behavioral model, with the patients medically monitored by their own physicians. Groups should consist of eight to ten individuals at the most and be either ongoing or time limited. Some MCOs will allow clients only a time-limited number of group sessions, so clients need to utilize group only when they need intensive booster sessions. I have had essentially the same eating-disorder group for ten years, with new members coming into it and leaving and old members returning whenever they need some extra help. In addition, I offer a free session for parents the first Monday evening of every month. Typically, once a year I send out a flyer advertising my group-treatment program to my primary referral resources: physicians, colleges, and high school guidance counselors. My groups include self-pay individuals as well as those who utilize their insurance benefits.

3. Other marketing activities my colleagues have developed include providing women's network lunches, in which therapists sit in and discuss such topics as eating-disorder prevention and mother-daughter relationships. One colleague offers twice a year free breakfast meetings/training to counselors and clergy.

4. Many practices are marketed using brochures that are sent to general practitioners, mental-health colleagues, local organizations, attorneys, former clients, and clergy. Most of the best professional brochures include some of the following elements: (A) Discussion of the benefits of their program, (B) Eye-catching headlines such as ARE YOU AFRAID OF EATING? WE WANT TO HELP, (C) Summary of what the program can accomplish rather than recital of credentials, (D) No commercial sales pitches, (E) Question-and-answer format and a list of the symptoms of eating disorders, (F) Photos of the therapists (one colleague includes the name and picture of his secretary so clients "know" the person to whom they will be speaking).

5. Eating-disorder specialists who are looking for extra job security may want to network with local intensive-outpatient programs and partial-hospitalization programs. Some may be open to the idea of contracting with an independent therapist to handle specialized groups like eating disorders that they are unable to handle in-house. One way to break into this market might be to offer a day-treatment group program. Calling directors of intensive outpatient treatment programs is a place to start.

6. The majority of my referrals come from physicians, and I work hard at maintaining this referral relationship by providing timely feedback. I prefer to send written progress notes, and I usually send a thank you as well as the first progress note immediately after the initial session. I always try to find out from each physician how they want follow-up handled. Some of my physician colleagues would rather have a monthly summary than receive weekly progress notes that add to the enormous paperwork they already have. Some prefer a phone call. Assess the best communication method for each physician, and also return the referral.

7. Always make sure all phone calls are instantly handled. We utilize a form that includes the date of the call, the time, initials of the person taking the call, caller's name and number, referral source, and what was done for the caller. Recently I decided to

do all of my own scheduling via a pager. For years I let secretaries handle this, but I now realize how much clients appreciate talking to the therapist. Doing my own scheduling allows me to have much more control over my practice as well as allowing me to take time off and away from the practice whenever I choose. One of the most important functions that my secretaries perform is confirming my appointments. Clients are asked during the initial session how they want us to handle this. My staff is trained precisely how to answer phone calls, and we avoid putting clients on hold. We also try not to let the phone ring more than a couple of times.

Breaking Free of Managed Care

As I write this chapter I am looking at the end of my career as it now exists and making a transition to semiretirement. If I was at the beginning of my career instead of the end, I would do everything I could to develop a third-party-free practice.

Psychologist Dana Ackley successfully transitioned his third-party-dependent practice to a private-pay practice. He utilized newsletters to referral sources writing about clinical issues such as school phobias, stressors of adolescence, and other clinically relevant topics. In his transition to private-pay practice he sent out one newsletter issue titled *Managed Care and Outpatient Therapy,"* in which he described the kinds of changes that were happening and the ways in which money drove managed care. The newsletter also described his dilemma of either cooperating or going out of business. The newsletter concluded with a description of private-pay therapy and its advantages, and immediately his referrals went up. From that time on he began to give clients two handouts, the first describing the pros and cons of using health insurance to pay for therapy, the second outlining payment plan options. Today his practice is 90 percent free of third-party payments.

Dr. Ackley cites three basic principles for making services attractive and/or high-priority to potential clients:

1. *Learn what feels urgent to people.* What do people want from us? For example, is there a need for an adolescent girls group that is food preoccupied? Is there a need for a therapy group for parents of eating-disordered children? Are there enough potential clients for an intensive one-day-a-week program? What services do the neighboring colleges and universities offer students with eating disorders? Who do they refer to in the community? Are there professionals who need training and/or supervision?

2. *Offer services that address these needs, let people know what we have to offer, and why it is worth their money and time to consult with us.* Ackley presents "marketing" as helping potential clients learn about the value and availability of services we can provide. This can be accomplished ethically and professionally. I would not be writing this book if I felt no one would buy it. In essence I am marketing my values, beliefs, and methods. If I wanted to seriously attract a self-pay clientele, I would cut prices and allow a 20 percent discount for those who would pay each week.

3. *Overcome the obstacles that keep people from seeking our services.* Dr. Ackley's problem-solving/skill-building model discusses everything from how to present your practice in the yellow pages to seminars, circulars, and brochures as ways of communicating with target groups.

12 .

Our Daughters, Ourselves

A LOOK TO THE FUTURE

OVER the past decade Bill and I became painfully aware of sex-role stereotyping and how it has kept women from realizing their full potential. Through our work we identified strongly with women's struggles against societal pressures. And observing these pressures on our own children reinforced our belief that today's parents and future parents must commit themselves to help young women achieve independent adulthood. Fathers must not protect their daughters from challenge and responsibility—recent studies of successful women have consistently revealed strong childhood relationships with fathers who encouraged risk taking, stamina, and strength of character rather than passivity and the traditional feminine role. And mothers must serve as powerful models for their daughters—the parent who shows rather than tells offers invaluable guidance.

However, this is not enough. In movies and on television, in magazine articles and advertisements, we are continually bombarded with unrealistic and unhealthy models of womanhood. Hundreds of thousands of young women strive for a feminine ideal that is nearly impossible to attain, and the ramifications add up to a major health threat. Several clinics now offer eating-disorder programs for girls as young as five and six! All over our country activists are willing to go to jail to save trees, whales, spotted owls, or mountain lions. Who is working to save our starving, dying girls?

The prevailing culture seems so dangerous to women that I actually feel relief that my own two daughters have produced sons instead of daughters.

Talking to our girls, instilling feminist values, and educating parents are all still *not enough* to offset the constant parade of anorexic models in the media. In the late 1960s a single model, Twiggy, ushered in cultural ideals of unnatural thinness. In the 1990s many of the most celebrated/emulated stars, including Calista Flockhart of *Ally McBeal,* Gwyneth Paltrow of *Shakespeare in Love,* and Courtney Cox of *Friends* look equally emaciated. When adolescent girls compare their own bodies to these women, it is not surprising that a majority will perceive themselves as fat, develop body hatred, and attempt to diminish themselves in a deadly competition to be the slimmest of all.

Hello?! Where have all the activists/feminists gone? Who is taking responsibility for what is happening to our girls? Recently, after three college students died, tremendous attention was given to male wrestlers' unhealthy "cut-weight" strategies for matches. Within a few weeks the NCAA purged these dangerous practices and issued new guidelines. Someone cared about these young men. Someone was speaking for them. Who was listening in 1997 when world-class gymnast Christie Henrich and ballet dancer Heidi Guenther, both age twenty-two, died of organ-system failure related to their struggles with anorexia nervosa?

Following the Littleton, Colorado, school massacre, calls went out to address the media's irresponsibility in marketing violence, and congressional meetings were held. There has been no such comparable demand to protect our growing girls from an irresponsible media marketing eating disorders. On a recent PBS program on eating disorders, Vidal Sassoon was asked whether he took any responsibility for eating disorders. The camera flashed to his models' dressing room where naked emaciated women, some who seemed to me disfigured by osteoporosis, were primping. He replied that he did not, adding that he viewed these current models as healthy and rather attractive.

Prevention programs will be ineffective until we confront and

alter what Mary Pipher labels as body destroying, media reinforcing, insane cultural values. We need more positive role models
such as Anita Roddick, the founder of The Body Shop, who sells
all-natural, environmentally sound beauty products. She found
the usual emaciated images of women unacceptable, abhorrent,
and damaging, and in her own advertising she has eliminated this
type of body ideal. *She is taking responsibility. She is speaking for our
girls.*

How about the rest of us? We need to boycott products, magazines, TV programs, and movies that reinforce this body type:
Speak up, act up, and advocate for our children. In 1997 I was glad
to read that feminist Naomi Wolf, author of *The Beauty Myth,* was
taking her "cause and anger" to Capitol Hill, calling for "a national program warning girls about the lethal consequences of eating disorders, on a par with programs to fight drug abuse." A year
and a half later I am unaware of any action taken to implement
such a program.

Responsibility rests with all of us to demand healthier models,
well developed and fit to replace the weak and emaciated ones
who convey the destructive, subliminal message: If you could lose
weight you would be perfect.

Models and actresses who are pressured to maintain unhealth-
ily slim bodies could begin to resist in concerted ways just as air-
line flight attendants successfully fought efforts to discriminate
against them in terms of age, marital status, and weight restrictions.
Corporations that market products to youngsters need to follow
the example of Anita Roddick. Editors of magazines and produc-
ers of films could help by refusing to hire models and actresses
who are emaciated. I truly believe images of healthier, more wom-
anly models and actresses who have curves could save lives.

Joan Ryan, in her book *Little Girls in Pretty Boxes* (1996), provides a scathing indictment of the coaches of elite athletes, accusing them of exploiting gymnasts and figure skaters and pushing
them into eating disorders, emotional breakdowns, and even death.
She calls for a serious reevaluation of what we're doing in this

country to produce Olympic champions. Dance and athletic coaches could exert their influence and become more responsible and informed about the physiological and psychological ramifications of eating disorders. If they knew about nutrition as well, they might recognize the potential damage resulting from misperceptions about body weight. For example, the historical ritual of weighing in before an audience can create anxiety, so the sensitive coach might recommend that an "overweight" child see a nutritionist or physician who could support and educate her in attempts at weight regulation. At the same time, the ill effects that dieting can have on performance and stamina need to be emphasized. Finally, the youngster should not be given any ultimatum about weight loss lest she resort to strategies like bulimia.

Schools, colleges, and universities have the power and the means to offset some of the more crippling effects of antifat attitudes. Health-education courses could routinely provide relevant reading material, guest speakers, and forums that might curtail and ultimately prevent the epidemic of eating disorders. For example, female students in elementary schools and junior and senior high schools, who represent a high-risk population, might be screened using a body cathexis test and questionnaire. Those with negative attitudes about their bodies could then be invited to participate in discussion groups with trained psychologists, nutritionists, and nurses. Such programs may prove to be essential since bulimia and anorexia at the elementary-school and high-school level are showing an appalling increase. (One survey published in the *Journal of the American Medical Association* [March 21, 1986] found that 13 percent of the 1,728 tenth-grade students polled reported purging behavior.) School systems need to take a serious look at emaciated teachers. It deeply angers me to hear my eight- or ten-year-old anorexic clients talk about wanting to look like their too-thin teachers. We would not allow these women to teach if they had an evident drug or alcohol problem; they would have to take a medical leave until they recovered. Why should eating disorders be treated differently?

A Model Program for Schools

Rebecca Axelrod, a recovered bulimarexic and an eating-disorders consultant, was very active in creating a good program in Meriden, Connecticut. When guidance counselors at the H. C. Wilcox Vocational Technical School became concerned about the increasing number of girls complaining about their weight and admitting to severe dieting practices, Rebecca was asked to speak about eating disorders and their effect on the body. After the lecture, several girls approached the counseling department, asking for help, voicing concerns about the abnormal eating patterns of their fellow students. The guidance department then realized there was a tremendous need for educational and remedial work. Rebecca was asked to form a group that would focus on body image, nutrition, and the dangers of dieting.

The eight girls chosen ranged from ages thirteen to seventeen. One was a former anorexic, four were bulimarexic, and the remaining three were chronic dieters with abnormal eating patterns. All were obsessed about getting fat and striving for the "perfect" body. This group met each week for one hour and began by assessing individual needs. Each girl was questioned about diet history, feelings about food, and her own body image. Based on these questions and individual evaluations, the following areas were covered during the school year:

1. Nutrition and health
2. Self-esteem and self-respect
3. Relationships with peers, family, and food
4. Myths related to dieting and weight
5. Body image and acceptance
6. Sexuality
7. Techniques for dealing with negative feelings and bad habits
8. Taking responsibility for oneself
9. Expectation levels and acceptance
10. Goal contracting and setting achievable goals

This group became a huge success with all participants. The bulimarexics ceased to binge, and the self-starving girls stopped dieting and starving and became obsessed, instead, with good nutrition. When the group began, Rebecca asked the girls to complete statements such as:

1. What I like best about myself is . . .
2. What I like least about myself is . . .
3. The best thing about being female is . . .
4. The worst thing about being female is . . .
5. I would like my body if . . .
6. The perfect body is . . .

Initially the answers to "The perfect body is . . ." went something like: "petite," "no more than 110 pounds," "thin, with a small waist, like a model's," "a size 5." At the end of the school year the responses were: "There is no such thing," "in proportion and if the person is happy with herself," "healthy," "the way you look at yours," "just the way God gave it to me."

These encouraging responses demonstrated that beliefs and habits can be modified by group cooperation and through guidance and education. Rebecca's program has now expanded to include other schools in Connecticut.

College Programs

Many colleges and universities have initiated preventive educational courses and treatment groups. At the University of North Carolina at Chapel Hill, students receive help at a drop-in center called the New Well. Here are some of the excerpts from their literature, offering target topics:

Nutrition Education for Bulimics: Has binge/purging been a problem for you? Learn how to eat sensibly and nutritiously while challenging the binge/purge dilemma.

Bet 'Ya Can't Eat Just One: Is your eating out of control? Be prepared to discuss compulsive eating . . . what it is, how to cope, and learn to set realistic management goals.

Eating on Target: Eating nutritiously at college is challenging. Find out how to plan and choose foods wisely—tips to assist your decisions.

Junkbusters: Are you a "fast-food fanatic" who depends on others to prepare your meals? If so, learn to develop a personal "junkbusting" program to assist you in making better choices.

At the University of Maryland Health Center, health educators, social workers, and nutritionists join together to provide comprehensive outreach programs for the prevention of eating disorders. This team routinely visits residence halls, sororities, and academic classes. Workshops such as "Food and Feelings" are offered every semester. All faculty and administrators receive a newsletter designed to help them become aware of these problems. Resident advisers (RAs) are trained to recognize eating disorders in their dorms. At Harvard, Eating Problems Outreach was instituted in order to provide a nonthreatening environment where women with eating problems could turn to peer counselors for help, support, and information. Counselors Toby Simon and Robin Rose developed Food Preoccupied Groups at Princeton for women who did not yet have serious eating disorders but might develop them in the future. These groups were designed to help students regulate their eating patterns. Colleges and universities need to take a hands-on, proactive approach and develop policies about self-endangerment.

I have consulted with the administration of Washington and Lee University in Lexington, Virginia, for several years on eating disorders and have rarely encountered a college that works so hard to help students remain in school while overcoming an eating disorder. They have an outreach program that insists on contracts regarding treatment signed by students, parents, and staff, then avails students of compassionate nutritional, medical, and psychological assistance. Dr. Jane Horton, director of Health Services, and Dr. Anne Schroer-Lamont, associate dean and counseling psychologist, have contributed the following details about their excellent program:

Eating disorders are managed at Washington and Lee University using a team approach. This approach is applied across all three phases of management: preventive/education, intervention/evaluation/on-campus treatment, and referral/off-campus treatment. Professional staff involved in these three phases include physicians and nurses at the Student Health Center, counselors at the University Counseling Service, the health educator, athletic training staff, and Student Affairs administrative staff. Students are trained and supervised by the professional staff in roles as peer helpers through peer counseling, student-athlete mentor, peer health education, and residence life programs.

Targets for prevention/education programs about eating disorders developed by professional staff include the student peer helpers noted above, Student Affairs staff, athletes and coaches, student organizations (e.g., sorority chapters, special interest organizations), student subpopulations such as the law school or the freshman class, and the general student body. Such programs include media campaigns, brochures, screenings, educational programs, and peer-led discussions.

Intervention strategies are presented to the campus in these various programs and print media. Professional staff will counsel friends or faculty/staff who are planning an intervention to maximize success in getting an individual in for evaluation. Evaluations may be initiated with either medical or counseling staff. The individual is then referred to the other service to complete the evaluation. Information from these evaluations is shared, with permission of the student, between the health and counseling services. Medical confidentiality of this information is maintained (with the exception of situations judged to require administrative involvement under the University's Policy on Self-Endangerment). The physicians and counselors meet twice monthly to review shared cases and communicate frequently as an individual treatment plan is being developed to make sure that treatment strategies, behavioral expectations, monitoring, and follow-up are consistent.

Washington and Lee has around-the-clock availability of health services on campus, with a nurse on duty and a physician and a professional counselor on call whenever school is in session. There is no limitation placed on student utilization of counseling or health services. This level of care is often not available at other institutions and helps us to continue on-campus treatment of students with serious eating disorders. Our incoming students are all expected to complete a health history, which specifically asks for any history of eating disorders. Students who acknowledge any such history are called in to meet with a physician in the Student Health Center during the first few weeks they are on campus. This visit serves to evaluate their current status, make them aware of campus support resources, and consider the need for ongoing treatment.

Referral off campus for further evaluation or treatment may be recommended or required, depending on the severity of the case. This referral may be to an eating disorders specialist, a psychiatrist, or another appropriate specialist. If such referral is required, the University will pay for the initial evaluation visit. The student is then responsible for the costs of ongoing off-campus care, including hospitalization if necessary. Records of a required evaluation are made available to the treating professionals at the University as part of the confidential medical record.

An Eating Disorder Therapy group meets weekly in the counseling service. Some students choose to attend this group instead of having individual counseling or in addition to their weekly individual appointment. The group members are very supportive of one another and provide an opportunity for women to discuss their personal problems with peers who have a higher level of understanding about the eating problems than their other peers have. The group remains open so that new members can join as the year progresses. Sometimes structured reading and discussions are planned, but more often the ninety minutes are open for any topic that the members want to address.

The University Health Educator is available to meet with students about their eating problems and helps them plan healthy eating choices within the on-campus eating establishments. First-year students are required to eat in the main dining hall, and therefore the health educator works with the dining hall manager to develop special privileges for students who are required to gain weight. Snack boxes are available along with special menu items, which can be ordered when the regular menu options would only cause one to binge and purge or to avoid eating altogether. Another service the Health Educator provides is to meet with the off-campus students with eating problems who are seeking recipes for healthier eating and/or vegetarian eating.

If a student does not cooperate with the treatment plan and continues to engage in self-endangering behavior, the professional staff will involve the Dean of Students. Under the University Policy on Self-Endangerment, the Dean of Students will require an assessment of the student's need for treatment and ability to continue at the University. At that point such an assessment will become a part of the student's administrative record rather than remaining in the confidential health record. Based on this assessment and in consultation with the professional staff, the Dean may . . . recommend a voluntary withdrawal from the University for medical reasons or may implement an administrative withdrawal if the student is felt to represent a serious health risk to self and fails to undergo the required evaluation or comply with recommended treatment. . . . When a student must leave campus to be hospitalized or to receive intensive out-patient care, the medical and psychological staff work with the Readmissions Committee to help plan for the return of the student.

As we can see from Washington and Lee's commitment to its students, some of the most effective psychotherapy for eating disorders is being offered on college campuses. Feminist consciousness-raising is often an integral component of treatment, and more female therapists are available. Equally important, the all-woman's group is not viewed with suspicion as a political forum but accepted as another support network outside of therapy. The emphasis on a sociocultural perspective within a short-term crisis intervention model allows women to depend on themselves and other women rather than reinforcing a years-to-treat individual pathology mentality.

Aggressive preventive and treatment programs that take into account the female experience are beginning to offer a welcome balance to the interpretation and treatment of eating disorders as practiced by a majority of male medical practitioners. William Davis, director of the Center for the Study of Anorexia and Bulimia, points out that "while there are many female therapists treating anorexia nervosa, the commonly acclaimed experts in the field—those who publish the most and therefore are most influential regarding treatment techniques—are almost all male." Fortunately the number of women therapists who treat eating disorders is increasing.

Public awareness of the destructive consequences of eating disorders has also increased. Eating disorder aid societies throughout the country have provided an effective means of support for desperate women, their parents, and other loved ones. They provide invaluable referral information, sponsor conferences, and groups where parents and loved ones can receive support and express their fears and pain. However, until very recently these groups have almost all focused on support rather than activism. Following the example of the highly successful National Breast Cancer Coalition, our girls need organizations devoted to the *politics of eating disorders* composed of feminists, educators, politicians, therapists, physicians, and parents of children with these problems.

Other successful models include the National Alliance for Research in Schizophrenia and Depression and the National Alliance for the Mentally Ill, grassroots organizations that raise millions of dollars for education, treatment, and research. In December 1998 a meeting was held in Washington, D. C., sponsored by the McKnight Academy for Eating Disorders to discuss methods to generate an eating-disorder bandwagon. The purpose of this meeting was to develop an alliance between eating disorder professionals, sufferers, and their families with the following goals:

1. Mobilize concerned citizens to advocate for attention from policy makers, the insurance industry, and the medical and scientific community.
2. Increase funding and support for new directions in research on causes, prevention and treatment.

The field desperately needs to recruit eager citizens who believe their participation will make a difference. Individuals and families who are interested should contact Dr. Walter Kaye, Director of Research, E-724 Western Psychiatric Institute and Clinic; 3811 O'Hara Street, Pittsburgh, PA 1521. Phone: 412-624-3507; fax: 412-624-6618,

Every eating disorder meeting/conference should provide sessions for training advocates similar to the National Breast Cancer Coalition Advocacy Training Conferences. They include plenary sessions, consisting of experts who provide reviews of recent activities in the following areas:

1. How to Build a Local Advocacy Network
2. Strategies for Effective Lobbying
3. Nuts and Bolts of Congress
4. Understanding the Media and Using the Media as a tool for activism.

Knowledge is power, and advocates can work on demanding action from members of Congress to make meaningful changes in scientific research and public policy in order to acquire federal funding for preventive programs in the schools.

Self-help groups have also been organized for women with eating disorders. Cross-country networks have been established, often with the guidance, leadership, and example of women who once struggled with and overcame these same problems. Through these kinds of supportive consciousness-raising experiences, women gain a more balanced perspective not only about their own bodies but about the stifling aspects of the role assigned to them by society.

Other self-help possibilities include Overeaters Anonymous, cited frequently by our clients as exceedingly helpful, and assertiveness-training courses. While these suggestions should not be thought of as substitutes for a well-conceived therapy, if women are motivated to change their behavior, the prognosis is good. Family doctors, endocrinologists, and nutritional counselors can help too.

For women who seek therapy, it would be wise to ask questions about the approach and philosophy of the therapist during an initial exploratory session. For instance, will the therapy focus on the present habitual response, with strategies for eliminating the eating disorder, or will it concentrate on past, underlying conflicts? Does the therapist advocate a long- or short-term treatment? Will the sessions be individual or utilize a group approach? Has the therapist been successful in treating eating disorders?

Once therapy is under way, progress should be evident in several weeks. If not, both client and therapist should reexamine mutual goals in order to establish the most effective strategies or to ascertain whether the particular therapist/client relationship should be continued.

THIS book has focused on the unique problems of girls and women who are expected to conform to cultural ideals no matter how devastating the consequences. Our society imprisons women in their bodies and terrorizes them with the threat of social rejection. Boys also suffer from socialization pressures, such as glorifying athletes— "the jocks." With both girls and boys subjected to deadly socialization rituals, clearly there is a need to unite in action to offer a future for *all* our youngsters in which they can feel safe and secure no matter who they are, what interests they have, or how they look.

Because of the overwhelming response I have received, I will continue to offer intensive weekend workshops for women struggling with bulimia four times a year at Wild Wind Farm. Those interested may write to me at 5931 Graysontown Road, Radford, VA 24141. Please enclose a self-addressed stamped envelope.

In the meantime here is a list of selected books and other resources that may prove helpful.

Chesler, Phyllis. *Women and Madness.* New York: Doubleday, 1972; paper, New York: Avon Books, 1973.

Dowling, Colette. *The Cinderella Complex: Women's Hidden Fear of Independence.* New York: Summit Books, 1981; paper, 1982.

Ehrenreich, Barbara, and Diedre English. *For Her Own Good: 150 Years of The Expert's Advice to Women.* New York: Anchor Books, 1979.

Freedman, Rita. *Beauty Bound.* Lexington: Lexington Books, 1986.

Friedan, Betty. *The Feminine Mystique.* New York: W. W. Norton, 1983; paper, New York: Dell, 1977.

Harris, Thomas. *I'm OK, You're OK.* New York: Harper & Row, 1969; paper, New York: Avon Books, 1973.

Norwood, Robin. *Women Who Love Too Much.* Los Angeles: J. P. Tarcher, 1985; paper, New York: Pocket Books, 1985.

Peele, Stanton, and Archie Brodsky. *Love and Addiction.* New York: Taplinger Publishing, 1975; paper, New York: New American Library, 1976.

Pipher, Mary. *Reviving Ophelia.* New York: Ballantine Books, 1994.

Polivy, Janet, and C. Peter Herman. *Breaking the Diet Habit: The Natural Weight Alternative.* New York: Basic Books, 1983.
Rivers, Caryl, Rosalind Barnett, and Grace Baruch. *Beyond Sugar and Spice: How Women Grow, Learn and Thrive.* New York: Putnam, 1979; paper, New York: Ballantine, 1981.
Russianoff, Penelope. *Why Do I Think I am Nothing Without a Man?* New York: Bantam, 1982; paper, New York: Bantam, 1982.
Ryan, Joan. *Little Girls in Pretty Boxes.* New York: Warner Books, 1995.
Sanford, Linda T., and Mary Ellen Donovan. *Women and Self-Esteem.* New York: Anchor Press, 1984; paper, New York: Penguin, 1985.
Vincent, L. M. *Competing with the Sylph: Dancers and the Pursuit of the Ideal Body Form.* New York: Andrews & McMeel, 1980; paper, New York: Berkley, 1981.
Wolfe, Naomi. *The Beauty Myth.* New York: William Morrow, 1991.

Eating disorder self-help books I particularly like are those written by Lindsey Hall and Leigh Cohn. They include:

Bulimia: A Guide to Recovery, new edition. Carlsbad, Calif.: Gurze Books, 1999.
Anorexia Nervosa: A Guide to Recovery. Carlsbad, Calif.: Gurze Books, 1998.
Self-Esteem: Tools for Recovery. Carlsbad, Calif.: Gurze Books, 1990.

Contact the publisher at Gurze Books, P.O. Box 2238, Carlsbad, CA 92018.

For managed-care strategies, I recommend:

Ackley, Dana C. *Breaking Free of Managed Care.* New York: The Guilford Press, 1997.
Psychotherapy Finances (newsletter), P.O. Box 8979, Jupiter, FL 33268, phone 800-869-8450.

New Harbinger Publications has published several workbooks dealing with anxiety and depression. The following ones are very useful:

Goodbye Good Girl. Clegg, Elten M., and Susan Swartz, 1998.
When Perfect isn't Good Enough. Antony, Martin M., Ph.D., and Richard P. Swanson, M.D., 1998.
The Worry Control Workbook. Copeland, Mary Ellen, M.S., 1998.
The Depression Workbook. Copeland, Mary Ellen, M.S., 1992.
Thoughts and Feelings: Taking Control of Your Moods and Your Life, Second Edition. McKay, Matthew, Ph.D., Martha Davis, Ph.D., and Patrick Fanning, 1998.

The following national nonprofit organizations offer help and support:

Academy for Eating Disorders
6728 Old McLean Drive
McLean, VA 22101
703-556-9222
www.acadeatdis.org

The Academy of Eating Disorders is an association of professionals that addresses effective treatment. It also focuses on prevention, advocates for the field, conducts research, and sponsors conferences.

American Anorexia/Bulimia Association
165 West 46th St. #1108
New York, NY 10036
212-575-6200
http://members.aol.com/AmanBu

A source of information: support groups, educational programs, professional programs and training. They also publish a quarterly newsletter.

National Association of Anorexia Nervosa and Associated Disorders
P.O. Box 7
Highland Park, IL 60035
708-831-3438
www.members.aol.com/anad20

This organization is known for its distribution of information, including lists of therapists and hospitals. They sponsor support groups as well as conferences and advocacy campaigns. A crisis hot line is also part of their agenda.

Eating Disorders Awareness and Prevention
603 Stewart St. #803
Seattle, WA 98101
206-382-3587
www.members.aol.com/edapinc/home.html

Focuses on (and sponsors) Eating Disorders Awareness Week in February, involving a network of state coordinators and educational programs.

International Association of Eating Disorder Professionals
427 Whooping Lane #1819
Altamonte Springs, FL 32701
800-800-8126
www.iaedp.com

This is a membership organization for professionals. It provides certification and education as well as local chapters, a newsletter, a monthly bulletin and an annual symposium.

National Eating Disorders Organization
6655 S. Yale Ave.
Tulsa, OK 74136
918-481-4044
www.laureate.com

The focus is on distribution of information and a newsletter. They hold an annual conference which focuses on prevention, education, research, and treatment referrals.

National Center for Overcoming Overeating
315 W. 86th St. #17B
New York, NY 10024
212-875-0442

Offices are located in New York, New England, Chicago, Houston, and Atlanta. They offer an educational and training organization dedicated to ending body hatred and dieting.

The following Web sites offer many alternatives for education, referral and self-help:

InnerSolutions
www.innersolutions.net

Loving, nondiet approach to healing, food, weight, and body-image issues

Gurze Books
www.gurze.com

Eating disorders resources and links to other sites

Something Fishy
www.something-fishy.com

Huge Web site with resources for eating disorders

Begin from Within
www.jfcs.org/bfw.html

Workshops and therapy groups in Northern California

Overeaters Anonymous E-mail group
www.hiwaay.net/recovery/

Eating Disorders-Food Addiction Resources
http://www.jps.net/Sunflake/ED.htm

Mirror-Mirror
http://www.mirror-mirror.org/eatdis

Optimal Eating
http://www.healthyeating.com/

Web site for therapists, professional workshops, and eating-disorders articles

Beat Bulimia
http://www.beatbulimia.com/

Contains a newsletter on bulimia, info on how a woman overcame bulimia

Males and Eating Disorder
http://www.primenet.com/danslos/male/home

Includes list and articles on the subject

Index